Medical World Walkabout
医療の世界を見渡そう

Naoko Ono

Makiko Ishida DaSilva

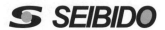

SEIBIDO

音声ファイルのダウンロード/ストリーミング

CD マーク表示がある箇所は、音声を弊社 HP より無料でダウンロード／ストリーミングすることができます。下記 URL の書籍詳細ページに音声ダウンロードアイコンがございますのでそちらから自習用音声としてご活用ください。

http://seibido.co.jp/ad609

はしがき

　近年の感染症の世界的な流行は、私たちにグローバル化をますます意識させることとなった。医療はグローバル化し、日本でも外国人を積極的に受け入れる医療機関が増えてきている。その他にも、日本の外国人人口が増えるに伴い、不慮の事故等で最寄りの医療機関を訪れる外国人数も増加することが予想される。特別な外国人の多い医療機関だけでなく、すべての医療機関に外国人対応の機会に備えることが有用であると考えられる。医療機関における外国人患者とのコミュニケーションでは、外国人受診者と日本人医療スタッフの文化的背景の違いから生じる行き違いに加えて、日本人スタッフの外国語能力が不十分な場合には誤解が生じやすい。さらに、言葉の壁が原因で、医療スタッフの治療に対する積極性に差が生じ健康格差につながる、という報告もある。このような背景の中でコミュニケーション不全や健康格差をなくすために、医療者が外国語の一つとして英語を学ぶ重要性はますます高まっている。

　本書は、医療英語を初めて学ぶ大学生を対象に、医療に関するさまざまな話題を満遍なく読む訓練と同時に、基本的な医療関連の背景知識を楽しみながら身に着けることを目的としたものである。また、各章の後半に Activity セクションを設けており、英文読解を起点として自分の意見を組み立てて英語にし、発信して、さらに仲間からのフィードバックを介して英語によるコミュニケーションを楽しめるようにした。ダウンロード可能な音声には、ネイティブスピーカーによる英語が収録されている。

　本書の作成に当たり、株式会社成美堂の佐野英一郎社長、松本健治氏、小亀正人氏、他の多くのスタッフの皆様にご指導、お力添えをいただいた。また、共著者との協力関係なしには本書を作成することができなかった。ほかにも本文の着想において貴重なご意見を賜った関係各位に深く感謝申し上げたい。

　本書が、医療のプロフェッショナルを目指す学生の皆さん、医学英語に興味を持ち学ぶ意欲のある学生の皆さんの学びの一助となることを願ってやまない。

2020 年 3 月 13 日
大野直子
ダシルヴァ石田牧子

本書の使い方

本書は、医療英語を初めて学ぶ学生を対象にしています。医療関連の比較的易しい文章の読解とその文章のテーマに関連するアクティビティーを通して、医療の背景知識を学び、楽しみながら英語でその情報を理解、発信、交換することを念頭に組み立てられています。

Pre-Reading Questions では、ペア（またはグループ）で本文の内容に関連する質問に答える形で、スピーキングやディスカッションを行います。本文を読む前のウォームアップの役割を果たします。

Vocabulary Check では、本文を理解する上で重要な、あるいはよく使われる単語の意味を確認します。

Reading Tips のある章では、リーディングの際に助けとなる基本的知識をトピックとして取り上げ、例文とともに紹介しています。Reading Tips の内容を意識しながら、次のステップに移ります。

Reading では、専門知識を必要としない幅広い医療関連の内容が比較的易しい英語で取り上げられています。本文の脇には、単語とその意味が掲載されてあり、必要に応じて単語の意味を確認しながら本文を読み進めます。ダウンロード可能な音声には、ネイティブスピーカーによる英語が収録されています。WPM も測ることができます。

Reading Comprehension では、問題形式で本文の内容理解を確認します。

Practice Conversation では、本文の内容に関連する医療現場の会話の例を聞き、実際に口に出して練習します。会話文には、本文中で扱った単語や、医療現場で頻回に使うフレーズが含まれているため、何度も口に出して練習してみましょう。ダウンロード可能な音声には、ネイティブスピーカーによる会話が収録されています。

Useful Expressions では、Practice Conversation 中で扱った、医療現場で役立つフレーズを再度確認します。

Writing Tips のある章では、簡単な文章作成の際に助けとなる基本的知識をトピックとして取り上げています。Writing Tips の内容を意識しながら、次のステップに移ります。

Activity では、本文の内容に関連のあるロールプレイ、ディスカッション、プレゼンテーションなどを通して、英語を使って楽しく意見やアイディアを発信したり交換したりする機会が設けられています。間違いを気にせずに、思っていることを英語で発信してみましょう。

Pre-test / Post-test

教科書の初めと終わりには、同じ内容のリーディングのテスト Unit が設けられています。Pre-test では英文読解の速さを測ることで、自分の今の単語力と英文をどれだけ速く正確に読む力があるかを測定しましょう。また、英語を学習する上で心がけようと掲げた目標と、自分を励ます一言を、英語で書いてみましょう。また、Post-test では単語力と英文を読む力をもう一度測定して、勉強を始める前と比べて上達しているか確認しましょう。Good Luck!

CONTENTS

人体各部位の用語

人体各部位の基本的な用語を覚えましょう。
下の英単語を手でかくして、日本語だけを見て英語が言えるようにしましょう。

人体各部位（前）

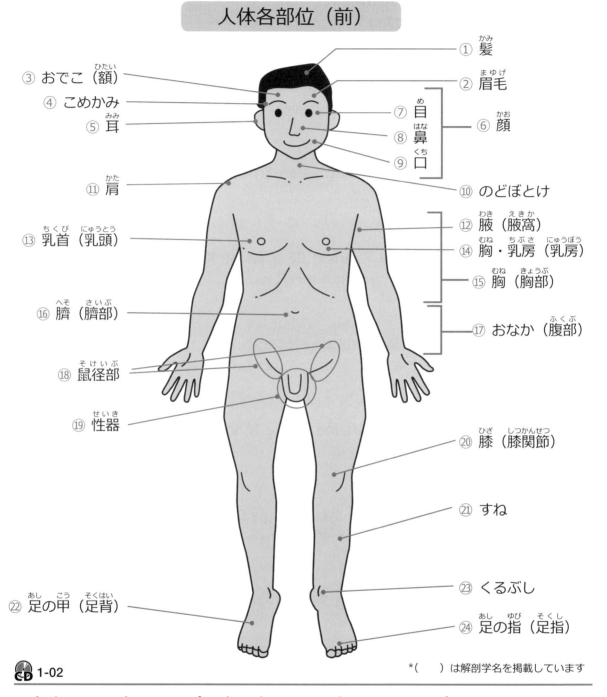

- ① 髪
- ② 眉毛
- ③ おでこ（額）
- ④ こめかみ
- ⑤ 耳
- ⑥ 顔
- ⑦ 目
- ⑧ 鼻
- ⑨ 口
- ⑩ のどぼとけ
- ⑪ 肩
- ⑫ 腋（腋窩）
- ⑬ 乳首（乳頭）
- ⑭ 胸・乳房（乳房）
- ⑮ 胸（胸部）
- ⑯ 臍（臍部）
- ⑰ おなか（腹部）
- ⑱ 鼠径部
- ⑲ 性器
- ⑳ 膝（膝関節）
- ㉑ すね
- ㉒ 足の甲（足背）
- ㉓ くるぶし
- ㉔ 足の指（足指）

🎧 CD 1-02

*（　）は解剖学名を掲載しています

① hair　② eyebrow　③ forehead　④ temple　⑤ ear　⑥ face　⑦ eye
⑧ nose　⑨ mouth　⑩ laryngeal / prominence / Adam's apple　⑪ shoulder
⑫ armpit / axilla　⑬ nipple　⑭ breast　⑮ chest　⑯ navel / belly button
⑰ stomach (abdomen)　⑱ inguinal region /groin　⑲ genitals / sex organ
⑳ knee (knee joint)　㉑ shin　㉒ instep　㉓ ankle　㉔ toe

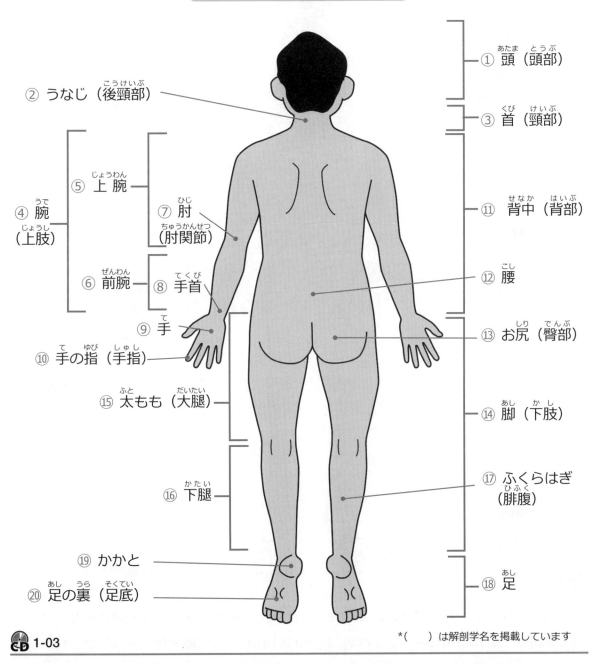

人体各部位（後）

② うなじ（後頸部<ruby>こうけいぶ<rt></rt></ruby>）

① 頭（頭部）
あたま とうぶ

③ 首（頸部）
くび けいぶ

⑤ 上腕
じょうわん

④ 腕
うで
（上肢）
じょうし

⑦ 肘
ひじ
（肘関節）
ちゅうかんせつ

⑥ 前腕
ぜんわん

⑧ 手首
てくび

⑨ 手
て

⑩ 手の指（手指）
て ゆび しゅし

⑪ 背中（背部）
せなか はいぶ

⑫ 腰
こし

⑬ お尻（臀部）
しり でんぶ

⑮ 太もも（大腿）
ふと だいたい

⑭ 脚（下肢）
あし かし

⑯ 下腿
かたい

⑰ ふくらはぎ
（腓腹）
ひふく

⑲ かかと

⑳ 足の裏（足底）
あし うら そくてい

⑱ 足
あし

🎵 1-03

*（　）は解剖学名を掲載しています

① head　② nape　③ neck　④ arm(upper extremity)　⑤ upper arm
⑥ forearm　⑦ elbow (elbow joint)　⑧ wrist　⑨ hand　⑩ finger
⑪ back　⑫ waist / hip　⑬ buttocks / bottom　⑭ leg (lower extremity)
⑮ thigh　⑯ lower leg　⑰ calf　⑱ foot　⑲ heel　⑳ sole

骨格各部位

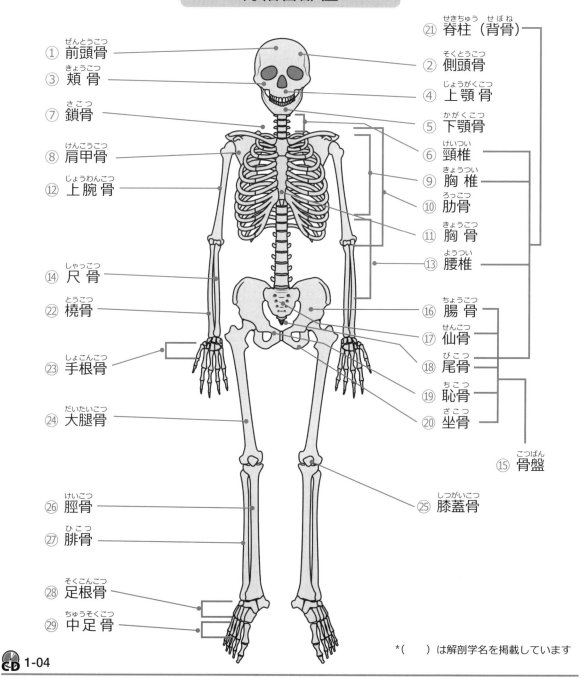

㉑ 脊柱（背骨）
せきちゅう せぼね

① 前頭骨
ぜんとうこつ

② 側頭骨
そくとうこつ

③ 頬 骨
きょうこつ

④ 上顎骨
じょうがくこつ

⑦ 鎖骨
さこつ

⑤ 下顎骨
かがくこつ

⑧ 肩甲骨
けんこうこつ

⑥ 頸椎
けいつい

⑫ 上腕骨
じょうわんこつ

⑨ 胸 椎
きょうつい

⑩ 肋骨
ろっこつ

⑪ 胸 骨
きょうこつ

⑬ 腰椎
ようつい

⑭ 尺 骨
しゃっこつ

⑯ 腸 骨
ちょうこつ

㉒ 橈骨
とうこつ

⑰ 仙骨
せんこつ

㉓ 手根骨
しゅこんこつ

⑱ 尾骨
びこつ

⑲ 恥骨
ちこつ

㉔ 大腿骨
だいたいこつ

⑳ 坐骨
ざこつ

⑮ 骨盤
こつばん

㉖ 脛骨
けいこつ

㉕ 膝蓋骨
しつがいこつ

㉗ 腓骨
ひこつ

㉘ 足根骨
そくこんこつ

㉙ 中足骨
ちゅうそくこつ

1-04

*（　　）は解剖学名を掲載しています

① frontal bone ② temporal bone ③ zygomatic bone /cheekbone
④ maxilla ⑤ mandible ⑥ cervical vertebrae ⑦ clavicle ⑧ scapula
⑨ thoracic vertebrae ⑩ rib ⑪ sternum ⑫ humerus ⑬ lumbar vertebrae
⑭ ulna ⑮ pelvis ⑯ ilium ⑰ sacrum ⑱ coccyx / tailbone ⑲ pubis
⑳ ischium ㉑ spine / backbone ㉒ radius ㉓ carpal bones
㉔ femur / thigh bone ㉕ patella / kneecap ㉖ tibia / shin bone ㉗ fibula
㉘ tarsal bone ㉙ metatarsal bone

Test Your Reading Skill : Team Medicine

チーム医療

あなたの今の単語力と、英文をどれだけ速く正確に読む力があるかを測定しましょう。

方法

1. 携帯電話や時計のストップウォッチ機能を起動します。
2. 先生の、「始め」という合図とともに読み始めましょう。
3. 読み終えたら、読むのにかかった時間を記録しましょう。
4. 本文の後の問題に答えましょう。
5. 最後に、もう一度最初から読んで、本文中のわからない単語に〇を付けてください。

 1-05

Toru was a naughty 10-year-old boy. One day, when he was climbing a tree with his friends, he saw a big insect crawling on it. He yelled and he fell down from the tree. His friends laughed at him, but gradually they became anxious because he did not open his eyes or even move. They called an ambulance, and paramedics rushed to the scene and took Toru to a nearby hospital. The paramedics quickly assessed the situation and determined the proper course of action. They realized his injuries were life-threatening, and they made sure that he was properly secured on a portable medical table stretcher which they then placed in the ambulance.

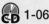 1-06

Toru was taken to the hospital, where he saw a physician and a nurse. The physician asked him what had happened. By that time, Toru had regained consciousness, but he was bleeding from his head, so a nurse took care of his wound. Toru seemed fine, but since he had fallen on his head from a height, the physician directed other medical professionals to conduct some examinations.

First, the radiology technician took an X-ray. It was very hard for Toru not to move. He was also shocked by the flash and the noise. Luckily, however, it was not painful.

He had blood taken and it was sent to the clinical technologist for analysis. The clinical technologist plays a crucial role in the process of detecting, identifying, and diagnosing illnesses and diseases. As a result of the X-ray and the blood test, no abnormality was found. To make sure, Toru was sent to an orthoptist for an eye test. Orthoptists help physicians to diagnose and treat a range of eye conditions. They carry out tests to help physicians to diagnose problems and determine appropriate treatment.

The results of the eye test were normal. Toru was discharged from the hospital but was told to visit periodically for physiotherapy. With the help of a physiotherapist, Toru will undergo some programs including working and moving his neck. A pharmacist will make sure if Toru understands the medications he takes.

🎧 **CD** 1-07

Can you count how many kinds of medical professionals helped Toru? In this passage, there were eight, but, many other care providers play a role in a patient's health.

Every day, these medical professionals work together and discuss each patient's progress. In this way, everyone on the care team can update the care plan along with the patient.

🎧 **CD** 1-08

Working as part of a team can come as something of a shock to experienced medical professionals. In their normal practice, they are accustomed to a strictly top-down approach, with the doctor making the decision and instructing a team of professionals to carry it out. It is only natural for experienced physicians to take a sense of pride in their knowledge, skills, and ability to set goals in patient care. But when working as part of a team, they must be prepared to set these factors aside and accept that the final decisions will be taken not individually but through consensus, the will of the majority, and deferring to those with greater expertise. But using multiple eyes can reveal many problems that could not be uncovered by a single eye. Everyone is a valuable member of the patient's care team. Respecting each other's opinions may be complex, but ultimately it is the most effective way to find the best care for the patient.

1 下記の表は、本文に出てきた職種をまとめたものです。空欄に適切な日本語を書き入れましょう。

職　種	仕 事 内 容
1.	
2.	
3.	
4.	
5.	
6.	
7.	
8.	

2 あなたが現在、1分間に読める文字数（WPM：words per minute）を求めましょう。

568語÷（読むのにかかった時間［秒］÷60）=（　　　　　　　　　）WPM

3 ○を付けた未知の単語を見てみましょう。1行に何個ありましたか。

4 読み方を自己評価しましょう。英文を読むときに、下記のことを頭に置いて読んでいましたか。
当てはまる場合には○を、当てはまらない場合には×を（　　　）に記入しましょう。

① 主語と述語を意識していた。　　　　　　　　　　　　　　（　　　）

② 最も重要な情報が何かを理解できた。　　　　　　　　　　（　　　）

③ 接続詞など、意味を左右する言葉に気を付けて読めた。　　（　　　）

5 英語を習う上で心がけようと考えた目標と、自分を励ます一言を、英語で書いてみましょう。

6 友人と目標を見せ合い、発表し合いましょう。

How Food Passes Through Our Body

体内を通る食べ物のゆくえ

私たちは、普段何気なく食事をしています。口から入った食べ物は、どのようにして体の中にとり込まれ、どこを通って体外に出るのでしょうか。食べ物の冒険に満ちた旅を見てみましょう。

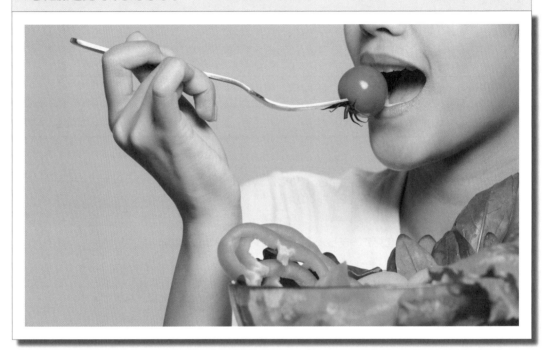

Pre-Reading Questions

ペアになり、以下について話し合いましょう。

List what organs food passes through in our body.

Vocabulary Check

次の単語とその定義を結びつけましょう。

1. swallow　　　　(a) a food that provides what is needed for one's body
2. nutrient　　　　(b) the system of organs responsible for breaking down of food
3. absorb　　　　 (c) to make food or drink go down your throat
4. digestive system (d) to take something in in a gradual way
5. beneficial　　　 (e) having a good effect

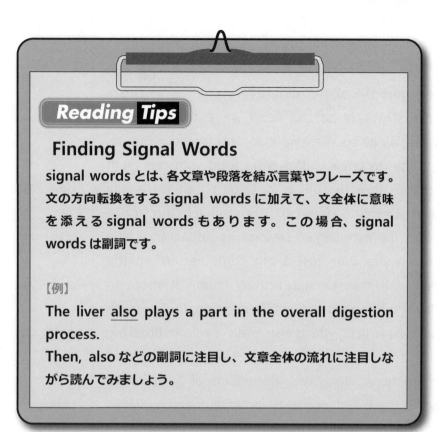

Reading Tips

Finding Signal Words

signal words とは、各文章や段落を結ぶ言葉やフレーズです。文の方向転換をする signal words に加えて、文全体に意味を添える signal words もあります。この場合、signal words は副詞です。

【例】

The liver <u>also</u> plays a part in the overall digestion process.

Then, also などの副詞に注目し、文章全体の流れに注目しながら読んでみましょう。

Reading

下記の英文を読みましょう。

1-09

Everyone knows which foods they like and which they find unappetizing. Most people are also well informed about which foods are beneficial for our health and which are not. But one thing that most people don't
5 know much about is what exactly happens to food once we take it inside our body.

In a sense, the digestive system housed inside our body operates in a similar way to an industrial refinery. Once the raw material—in this case food—enters the system,
10 it is subjected to a series of processes to separate what is useful from what is useless. The useful substances are then put to work to sustain the body's various functions

unappetizing ／おいしくない

industrial refinery ／産業用製油所

15

while the waste material is stored and expelled.

 1-10

The main purpose of the digestive system is to break down the structure of the food we eat. The whole process begins as soon as we put food into our mouth, and we begin to chew it. We grind food with our teeth and moisten it with saliva so that it can be easily swallowed, traveling down to the stomach through a tube called the esophagus. Despite its appearance, the stomach is more than just a big container. When the food reaches it, the stomach actively churns it about to break down the food structures. In addition, the stomach produces gastric acid, which also plays a role in breaking down food and killing bacteria. The tumbling and churning motions, along with the effects of gastric acid, lead to the release of nutrients, proteins, carbohydrates, and fats from the food we have ingested.

saliva ／唾液

esophagus ／食道

churn ／かき回す

gastric acid ／胃液

carbohydrate ／炭水化物

 1-11

On the next stage of its journey through the body, food enters the small bowel, a 7-meter-long tube tucked up inside of us. This is the place where nutrients from the food begin to be absorbed. The walls of the small bowel are lined with frond-like structures call villi, which increase the surface area for absorbing these nutrients. In between the villi are pits or crypts, where new cells that line the gut are produced. Food moves along this tube as the result of a wave-like motion called peristalsis. As it does so, it is broken down even further by the action of various enzymes.

frond-like ／葉っぱのような

villi ／絨毛

crypt ／地下室

gut ／消化管、腸

peristalsis ／蠕動(ぜんどう)運動

enzyme ／酵素

The liver also plays a part in the overall digestion process, producing bile, which helps fats to break down and be absorbed.

bile ／胆汁

 1-12

In the next stage, food passes through the large bowel, a

tube that is much wider than the small bowel and has no villi. Like the rest of the gut, its lining is covered in mucus, but rather than one layer, as is the case elsewhere, it has two layers, an inner and an outer, which are
5 important in maintaining a healthy gut. The inner layer prevents harmful bacteria from passing through the gut barrier, while the outer layer provides a suitable environment for beneficial bacteria to live. The large bowel also helps to absorb excess fluid, so that the waste
10 material can solidify into stool further down the bowel. In addition to this, it also contains literally trillions of bacteria—as many as ten times the number of cells in the rest of our body—which help to digest food and are a source of essential vitamins and other nutrients.

15 The final stage of the process is reached after the food has been digested. Any solid material remaining is excreted from the body as waste in the form of feces, whose distinctive odor is a result of bacterial action.

lining ／（胃の）内側
mucus ／粘液

stool ／便

WPM 580語÷（読むのにかかった時間[秒]÷60）＝（　　　　　）WPM

Reading Comprehension

下記の表は、本文に記された食物の通る器官をまとめたものです。（　）に適切な日本語を書き入れ、役割または特徴を書きましょう。

食物が通る器官 （順番に）	役割または特徴
esophagus （食道）	口から食べた食物、飲み物がここを通って胃に送られる。
stomach (1.　　　　)	
small bowel (2.　　　　)	
large bowel (3.　　　　)	
直腸→肛門	残りの水分が搾り取られたかすが、便となって体外へ出ていく。

Practice Conversation

受付と検査室での会話を聞いて、空欄にあてはまる語句を記入しましょう。
答えを確認した後、ペアになって会話を練習しましょう。

Nurse: Good morning. **May I help you?**

Patient: Good morning. I have an appointment at 10 o'clock.

Nurse: **May I have your name please?**

Patient: My name is John Brown.

Nurse: Yes, Mr. Brown. We've already received your information from your doctor. I have a few questions for you. **Can you please follow me this way?**

Patient: Sure. (They move to an exam room)

Nurse: Have you had any major surgery* before?

Patient: Yes, I had my [1.   ] taken out when I was 18.

Nurse: I see. Also, do you have any family history* of cancer?

Patient: Yes. My father had cancer of the [2.   ] a few years ago. It was treated successfully. This is one of the reasons that I'm really interested in [3.   ] the test [4.   ].

Nurse: I understand. We [5.   ] be able to look at the [6.   ] of the gut closely under the scope today.

Patient: That would be great....although I feel a bit sick to my [7.   ]. I guess I'm a bit nervous.

Nurse: I see. Most people feel nervous, and that's normal. I hope that the medication helps you [8.   ] the procedure. Is there anything that I can do for you?

Patient: No, I think I just need a moment to sit and relax. Thanks for asking.

Nurse: Sure. The doctor will be with you shortly.

*surgery 手術 *family history 家族歴

Useful Expressions

- **May I help you?** (どうなさいましたか？)

- **May I have your name please?** (お名前をお伺いしてもよろしいでしょうか。)

- **Can you please follow me this way?** (こちらへどうぞ。)

Activities

人間が食べ物を食べた場合には、上記の英文のような経路をたどりますが、別の生き物の場合は別の経路をたどったり、人間にはある内臓がなかったりします。人間以外の生き物のうち、内臓の構造が人間と大きく異なる生き物を2つ挙げて、その特徴をわかる範囲で英語で書いてみましょう。

Name of the creature	Characteristics

▶作文したことを、グループで発表しましょう。クラスメイトが発表したら、それに対して英語で一言意見を言いましょう。

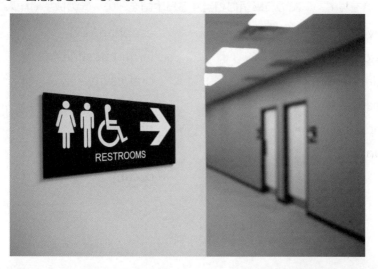

主な人体の器官

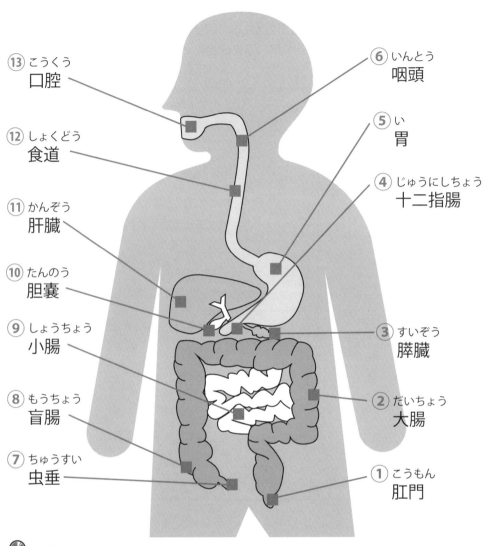

⑬ こうくう 口腔
⑫ しょくどう 食道
⑪ かんぞう 肝臓
⑩ たんのう 胆嚢
⑨ しょうちょう 小腸
⑧ もうちょう 盲腸
⑦ ちゅうすい 虫垂
⑥ いんとう 咽頭
⑤ い 胃
④ じゅうにしちょう 十二指腸
③ すいぞう 膵臓
② だいちょう 大腸
① こうもん 肛門

1-15

▶イラストを見て、下記の英単語に相当する日本語を、①〜⑬の数字で記入しましょう。

liver	( )	esophagus	( )
stomach	( )	large intestine	( )
duodenum	( )	oral cavity	( )
pancreas	( )	gallbladder	( )
appendix	( )	pharynx	( )
anus	( )	small intestine	( )
		cecum	( )

Coping with Cancer: Five Stages of Grief

がんと生きる：グリーフの5段階

重い病と診断された人の心の中は、どのようになっているのでしょうか。一度はショックを受けると思いますが、やがて患者は立ち直り、社会生活を再開する心の状態まで立て直します。このような患者の心の動きを研究した研究者が、病気に対する受容の過程を提示しました。本章では、各過程での心の動きや、どのようにして心を立て直して社会復帰していくのかを見ていきましょう。

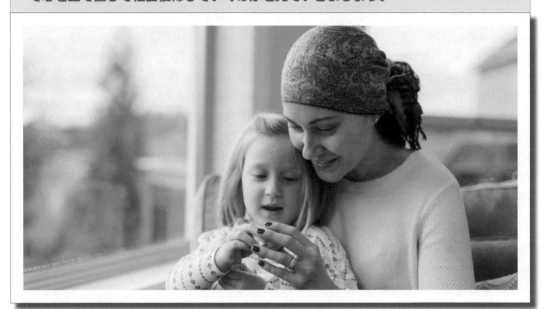

Pre-Reading Questions

ペアになり、以下について話し合いましょう。

How would you feel if you were diagnosed with an unexpected disease?

How would you cope with it?

Vocabulary Check

次の単語とその定義を結びつけましょう。

1. diagnose	(a) the refusal to accept a reality
2. denial	(b) the state of feeling without hope
3. bargaining	(c) to confirm the cause of a problem from the symptoms
4. depression	(d) agreement that something is right
5. acceptance	(e) discussions in order to reach agreement

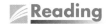
Reading

下記の英文を読みましょう。

CD 1-16

How would you react if you were unexpectedly diagnosed with a serious illness? How would you expect medical professionals and family members to treat you?

Dr. Elisabeth Kubler-Ross, an American psychiatrist who
5 has worked extensively with terminally ill patients, formulated a five-stage process that such people typically go through. The first stage is denial, in which the patient refuses to accept the diagnosis. This is followed by anger, when the patient thinks "Why me?" Then comes the
10 bargaining stage, when the patient wants help in exchange for doing something. The fourth stage is depression, while the fifth stage is acceptance, in which the patient comes to terms with the situation and tries to regain control over his or her life. Let's see how this
15 pattern applies in a real-life situation.

anger ／怒り

CD 1-17

Yoko was a 35-year-old company employee. She had been married for 10 years and was thinking of having a child. One day as she was taking a shower, she felt a sensation like a stone rolling inside her right breast. It
20 wasn't painful, so she ignored it. However, her mother was concerned and advised her to get it checked out at a hospital, where she was diagnosed with early-stage breast cancer.

company employee ／会社員

sensation like a stone rolling ／ごろごろする ような感触

early-stage ／早期の

breast cancer ／乳がん

In mid-career and with plans to start a family, Yoko
25 experienced the news as a powerful blow. She felt desperate. She refused to accept that she had cancer and went out drinking every night in an attempt to forget about it.

desperate ／絶望的

Eventually, Yoko told her boss and her co-workers about
30 the diagnosis. After a few weeks, she tried to calm down, but she found she couldn't suppress her anger at the unfairness of her condition. Different thoughts ran through her head. Why did I get breast cancer when I'm only in my 30s? Why me, not other people like my
35 colleagues A and B, who are unpleasant people and not

co-worker ／同僚

calm down ／落ち着く

suppress ／抑え込む

good at their jobs? And why now? It wouldn't be so bad if I had already had a child and the child was grown. I might have to have my right breast surgically removed, and the anti-cancer drugs will probably make my hair fall
5 out. What did I do to deserve this?

Yoko's physician listened carefully to her as she explained her feelings. In order to preserve her fertility, oncologists, obstetricians, and gynecologists worked together using the latest technology. Breast reconstruction surgery was
10 recommended to eliminate her sense of loss. When the course of anti-cancer drugs was over and hormone therapy started, Yoko decided to commit to medical care and do her best to make the treatment effective. But at this stage, she became anxious and wanted to do
15 whatever she could to suppress the cancer. She decided to adopt a strict vegetarian diet centered on brown rice, perhaps believing that she would be able to control her illness by eating healthy yet unappetizing food. However, there was no medical basis for this approach, and her
20 doctor persuaded her to go back to eating the foods she liked.

🎧 1-18

Hormone therapy was harder than Yoko had expected. Like chemotherapy, the first kind of treatment she received, it is not over in a few months but is a long-
25 term battle. The medication also had side effects and she suffered serious depression. After five years of treatment, she would be in her 40s, and her age might prevent her from having a child. She thought the inability to conceive would devalue her as a person. She also thought that if
30 her life had no meaning, it would be better for her to disappear, and she even contemplated committing suicide by throwing herself in front of a train. After she consulted her doctor, it was decided to cut down on her medication to mitigate this depression, which is a known
35 adverse effect of the treatment.

On the day Yoko received her final dose, her doctor told her that the main thing was to forget about the cancer and get on with her life. Now, 10 years after the treatment, she has heeded the doctor's advice and does
40 not think about the cancer as she goes about her daily activities. She even has a two-year-old son by her side.

anti-cancer drug ／抗がん剤

physician ／医師
fertility ／妊孕性(にんようせい：妊娠できること)
oncologist ／腫瘍内科医
obstetrician ／産科医
gynecologist ／婦人科医
reconstruction ／再建
eliminate ／除去する

brown rice ／玄米

persuade ／説得する

chemotherapy ／化学療法
side effect ／副作用

She had friends of her age who suffered from cancer but relapsed and died. When she thinks about them, she wants to appreciate the time she has been given. 🎧 1-19

relapse ／再発する

appreciate ／享受する

The five stages of acceptance are not always as neatly divided as they are with Yoko. Sometimes people flip back and forth between them. It is therefore a good idea for medical professionals and family members to keep a close eye on what patients are feeling so that they can help them feel better and live their lives with as much satisfaction as possible.

back and forth ／前後する

WPM 788語÷（読むのにかかった時間［秒］÷60）＝（　　　　　　　）WPM

▨ Reading Comprehension

下記の表は本文の内容をまとめたものです。（　）に入る適切な英単語を語群から選び、必要な場合は適切な形に変えて書き入れましょう。

denial	The first (1.　　　　　) to a terminal illness is to (2.　　　　　) the reality of the situation. The patient refuses to accept the diagnosis. This is a normal response to strong emotions.
anger	Once you return to reality, you might become angry. This is a common stage where you think "Why me?". The anger may be (3.　　　　　) at friends, family, and co-workers. We know these people are not to be (4.　　　　　). Emotionally, however, we may (5.　　　　　) them for causing us pain.
bargaining	When something bad happens, we might think, "If you (6.　　　　　) me, I will never eat my favorite food again." This is bargaining. You are so eager for your life to get back to normal. This is a kind of (7.　　　　　) to protect us from the (8.　　　　　) reality.
depression	Depression is a commonly accepted form of grief. In this stage, you might (9.　　　　　) from life and feel weak. The world might seem too much and too hard for you to face. You might even experience (10.　　　　　) thoughts such as "My life has no meaning; it would be better for me to disappear."
acceptance	In this stage, your emotions may begin to be (11.　　　　　). It's not a good thing, but it's something you can live with. It is a time of (12.　　　　　). You understand your previous life can never be (13.　　　　　), but you move, grow, and evolve into your new reality. You want to appreciate the time you have been given.

語　　群
stable / deny / resent / heal / withdraw / react / aim / adjust / defend / fall / notice / blame / pain / suicide / replace

◢ Practice Conversation 1-20

カウンセリング室での会話を聞いて、空欄にあてはまる語句を記入しましょう。
答えを確認した後、ペアになって会話を練習しましょう。

Clinical Psychologist*: I heard from your doctor that you've been feeling much better since the last time. How are you feeling today?

Patient: I feel relieved that I was able to finish everything that my [1.   ] recommended.

Clinical Psychologist: I see.

Patient: It's not been easy for me. Looking back, I think I was suffering more [2.   ] my depression than anything else.

Clinical Psychologist: Yes, I remember.

Patient: First I was so angry with myself and everybody else. I was [3.   ] denial. Then I was going back and [4.   ] between feeling [5.   ] and hopeful. Sometimes I felt so depressed that I thought this whole process was not even worth [6.   ].

Clinical Psychologist: It must have been very difficult for you.

Patient: Yes, it was. Remember I was crying all the time? Without all of you, I wouldn't have been able to [7.   ] it.

Clinical Psychologist: I'm glad I was able to support you in this process. Well, this is our last meeting until the next follow-up in a few months. Is there anything that you would like to address this time?

Patient: No. Thank you so much for always having [8.   ] there for me since day one.

Clinical Psychologist: **It's been my pleasure. Please give my regards to** your family.

Patient: I will.

Clinical Psychologist: **Please take care**.

*clinical psychologist 臨床心理士

Useful Expressions

- **It's been my pleasure.**（どういたしまして／お役に立てて光栄です。）
- **Please give my regards to....**（〜［人］にどうかよろしくお伝えください。）
- **Please take care.**（お気をつけてください／お大事になさってください。）

Writing Tips

Expressing Your Opinion, Part 1

あるテーマに対して、自分なりの意見を表現することは、慣れていないとなかなか難しいものです。日本語で思い浮かんだ意見を正確に翻訳するのは至難の業です。まずは、知っている英単語を組み合わせ、(S)(V) の幹を作り、その後必要に応じて枝葉（修飾）を加えましょう。以下は意見の述べる際に便利な表現です。

【例】

My view is that..., I believe that..., In my opinion...,
It is my impression that..., My opinion is that...,
I'm under the impression that...

Activities

病気の人に声をかけることは、一般に難しいと言われます。その人の悩みや心の状況に合わせた言葉を選ぶことが難しいからです。しかし、本章で学んだ受容の 5 段階のどの段階にいるかを見ることは、かける言葉を考えるうえでヒントになります。以下のシナリオについて考え、英語で述べましょう。

> **シナリオ：**あなたの友達が、早期の胃がんと宣告を受けました。将来起業を目指して熱心に働いていた彼は、とても落ち込んでやる気をなくし、仕事をやめたいとさえ言っています。あなたは彼に、何とかして治療と人生に前向きになってほしいと考えています。

State the problem （友達の悩みと、受容のどの段階にいるかを述べましょう）

_____

_____

_____

State your opinion （あなたがかけたいと思った言葉を述べましょう）

_____

_____

_____

Support your opinion （その言葉がふさわしいと思った理由を述べましょう）

- _____

- _____

- _____

Restate your opinion （あなたの提案、結論を再度述べましょう）

_____

_____

_____

▶クラスメイトに向けて、あなたの提案をプレゼンテーションしましょう。
　プレゼンテーションを聞いたクラスメイトは、提案に対して自分の意見を述べましょう。

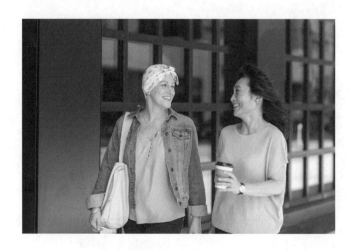

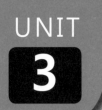

UNIT 3

Where Medicine Meets Religion

医療と宗教の出会うところ

診察を受ける際に、あなたの宗教を尋ねられたことはありますか。現代医学と宗教は一見すると接点がないように思えますが、特に海外の診療場面では自分の属している宗教や信条について聞かれることがよくあります。それは、宗教によっては、特別な注意を必要とする医療行為があるからです。その例を見てみましょう。

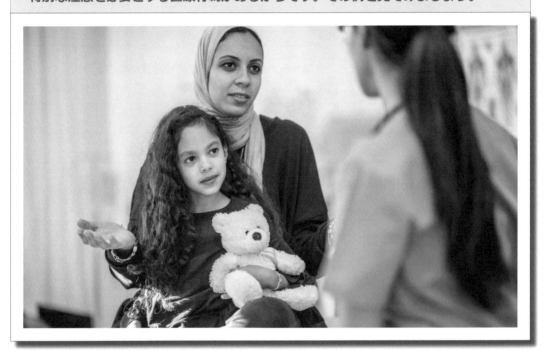

Pre-Reading Questions

ペアになり、以下について話し合いましょう。

Can you list some of the major religions of the world today?

Vocabulary Check

次の単語とその定義を結びつけましょう。

1. sacred   **(a)** a series of actions done in a certain way
2. define   **(b)** a part of a whole
3. procedure   **(c)** to give the meaning of a word or phrase
4. strict   **(d)** being regarded with great respect by a particular religion
5. component   **(e)** following rules or beliefs exactly

Reading Tips

Finding S and V

複雑な文章を読んでいるときに、主語がどれなのか迷ってしまうことはありませんか。(S) は主に「誰が (は)」「何が (は)」「〜することが (は)」「〜なことが (は)」という意味の語で、その後ろに (V) が続くという特徴があります。下の例文の (S) の候補は下線部ですが、どちらが (S) かわかりますか。

【例】

Because some medical procedures are invasive, clinical settings are some of the most intriguing settings when it comes to religion.

ここでは、接続詞がヒントになります。接続詞 because から始まる文は付け足し説明に過ぎず、幹となる文の settings が (S) であることがわかります。

Reading

下記の英文を読みましょう。

🎧 1-22

Our amazing, intricate body is regarded as sacred in many cultures and religions of the world. Treating a physical body in a certain way is often extremely important in many different beliefs. Many religions have
5 instructions for believers to keep themselves "clean" from whatever is defined as "unclean." Medicine often involves putting something into someone's body, whether in the form of pills, injections, IV drips, blood transfusions, or medical devices like pacemakers. Because of the invasive
10 nature of modern medical procedures, clinical settings are some of the most intriguing settings when it comes

intricate ／複雑な

injection ／注射
IV drips ／静脈点滴
blood transfusion ／輸血
invasive ／侵襲的な
intriguing ／興味をそそる

to religion.

 1-23

One of the most common religions in Asia is Islam. The Islamic faith has about 1.6 billion believers, nearly a quarter of the entire world population. More than 5 60 percent of Muslims are found in Asia, and about 20 percent in the Middle East and North Africa. [1] Every year in fall, millions of people from over 180 countries leave their homes and head for Mecca in Saudi Arabia for an Islamic pilgrimage called Hajj. As a part of their 10 preparation for this once-in-a-lifetime pilgrimage, they all need to receive certain types of medical care in order to take part in it. Can you guess what that would be?

pilgrimage ／巡礼

1-24

Due to extremely crowded conditions during Hajj, meningitis outbreaks have happened multiple times in 15 Saudi Arabia, affecting thousands of people. Meningitis is a serious infectious disease, which is typically accompanied by headache, fever, and stiffness of the neck, and spreads through contact with respiratory secretions. The disease can progress rapidly and can be fatal in up to 20 percent 20 of cases even with antibiotic treatment. [2] Meningitis occurs worldwide, but it is known to occur much more frequently in what is called the "meningitis belt" of sub-Saharan Africa as well as Saudi Arabia during the Hajj season. [3] Now, people traveling to Mecca during Hajj 25 are required by the Saudi Ministry of Health to receive a meningitis vaccination before entering the country. The requirement is so strict that people cannot get a visa unless they are vaccinated. [4]

meningitis ／髄膜炎

respiratory ／呼吸器の
secretion ／分泌物
fatal ／致命的な
antibiotic ／抗生物質の

sub-Saharan ／サハラ
以南の

vaccination ／予防接種

1-25

Vaccines, known to improve immunity to certain diseases, 30 not only contain weakened or dead microorganisms but also toxins that the organisms produce, certain types of proteins, and other things like preservatives. In the

immunity ／免疫
weakened ／弱毒化し
た
microorganism ／微生
物
preservative ／保存料

manufacturing process, some vaccines require components from animals such as chickens, cows, or pigs. Meningitis vaccines may not be exceptions, and this is what creates a dilemma for those who want to take part in Hajj.

🎧 1-26

5　As many people know, Muslims regard pigs as "unclean" and avoid pig-derived foods and products. Although they need to receive the meningitis vaccine, they face a conflict between medical and religious requirements. Some Muslim communities do not consider the vaccine

10　an issue at all. Others may be more circumspect. If an individual is experiencing the dilemma, one of the things he or she can do is to consult with his or her religious leader about different brands of meningitis vaccines. Some groups may officially approve a certain brand

15　because its manufacturer claims that its vaccines are free of pig gelatin or other pig products. Other groups may only provide some information and leave the decision up to individuals. Whatever the dilemma might be in a situation where medicine meets religion, the most

20　important thing may be to respect and support the individual's decision based on his or her belief.

derive ／〜から由来する

circumspect ／慎重な

approve ／承認する

1. Islam in Asia: Diversity in Past and Present, Cornell University, 2017
2. Traveler's Health Meningococcal Disease, Centers for Disease Control and Prevention, 2017
3. Meningococcal Disease in Other Countries, Centers for Disease Control and Prevention, 2019
4. Health Requirements and Recommendations for Travelers to Saudi Arabia for Hajj and Umrah, Saudi Arabia Ministry of Health, 2018

WPM 557語÷（読むのにかかった時間[秒]÷60）＝（　　　　　　　）WPM

Reading Comprehension

本文の内容を基に、下記の英文の（　）に入る適切な英単語を語群から選び記入しましょう。

1. Clinical settings can be some of the most intriguing settings when it comes to religions because modern medicine has an (1.   ) nature.

2. Visitors to Mecca during the Hajj season need to (2.   ) a meningitis vaccination.

3. Some Muslims are concerned that meningitis vaccines may contain animal (3.   ), and this creates a dilemma.

4. One can (4.   ) with one's religious leaders about different brands of vaccines.

5. Some groups may officially (5.   ) a certain brand of vaccine.

6. It is important to respect and support the individual's decision based on his or her (6.   ).

語　　群
circumspect / approve / belief / reject / microorganism / immunity consult / components / receive / invasive / collect / sacred / manufacture

Practice Conversation

🎧 1-27

病室での会話を聞いて、空欄にあてはまる語句を記入しましょう。
答えを確認した後、ペアになって会話を練習しましょう。

Nurse: Nice to meet you, Ms. Sari. I heard from the staff that you are from Indonesia.

Patient: Yes. I'm a bit nervous [1.   ] in a hospital for a few days. I just moved to Japan a couple months ago.

Nurse: I understand. We need to give you [2.   ] [   ] for a few days. I hope that the [3.   ] will work well and you feel better soon.

Patient: I hope so, too.

Nurse: While staying in the hospital, is there anything you can't eat for [4.   ] reasons?

Patient: I'm a [5.   ], so I can't eat pork. I also follow other [6.   ] rules during Ramadan*, which is starting in a week.

Nurse: **Can you tell me more about that?**

Patient: During Ramadan, I must not eat or drink during the day.

Nurse: You should be able to go home by [7.   ], but let me check what the doctor says about not [8.   ] meals regularly during Ramadan.

Patient: Will you? It's important for me.

Nurse: Of course. **I'll be right back.**

*Ramadan 断食月

Useful Expressions

🎵 1-28

• **Can you tell me more about that?**（もう少し詳しくお話しいただけますか。）

• **I'll be right back.**（すぐに戻ります。）

Activities

あなたが知っている限りの宗教を挙げ、それらの英語名を調べてみましょう。

-
-
-

-
-
-

▶ペアまたはグループになり、挙げられたリストを共有しましょう。その中から一つを選び、医療の場でどのような宗教的配慮 (religious considerations) が必要となりうるか調べ、下の枠内に英語で記入しましょう。

選んだ宗教の名称：
医療における宗教的配慮：

▶下の枠内の表現を参考にしながら、調べたことを英語でまとめ、クラスで発表しましょう。

> They believe that ….,They prefer …., It is important for them to …,
> We need to be careful not to …, We should ask their permission when …,
> We should avoid …, We need to pay attention to …

In our group, we looked at religious considerations for _____
(宗教の英語名) in medical settings.

_____

_____

_____

_____

_____

_____

_____

_____

_____

Thank you for listening. Do you have any questions?

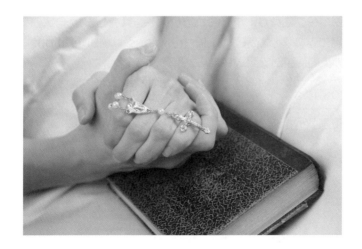

Before Calling It Malpractice

それって医療ミス？

十分に注意して車を運転しても、ある一定の確率で事故が起きてしまうように、医療現場においても残念ながら一定のリスクが伴います。よく耳にする「医療ミス」は、世間一般の人が思うほど単純な事柄ではありません。医療を受ける際に起こりうる有害な事象を理解する上で大切な概念について見てみましょう。

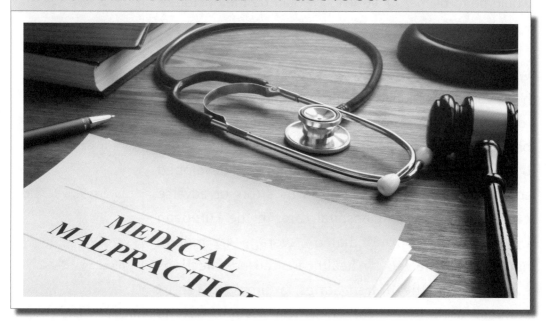

Pre-Reading Questions

ペアになり、以下について話し合いましょう。

How can you lower the risk of a driver getting into a car accident, besides the driver just being careful?

Vocabulary Check

次の単語とその定義を結びつけましょう。

1. prescribe | (a) to claim that someone is responsible for a fault
2. blame | (b) not able to be predicted
3. grasp | (c) a secondary condition making an already existing problem worse
4. complication | (d) to authorize the use of medicine
5. unpredictable | (e) to understand fully

◢ Reading

下記の英文を読みましょう。

🎧 1-29

Let's say you were prescribed a medicine. You then had to go to an emergency room later because you developed a rash all over your body after taking it. Who would be to blame? Of course, it would be the doctor...or
5 would it?

When things do not go as expected in medicine, healthcare professionals on the frontline are most likely to be the ones patients blame. This is understandable because medical accidents can be life threatening. It has
10 been estimated that one in 10 patients in developed countries experience harm caused by errors or adverse events while receiving hospital care. In the European Union, it was reported that on average 4.1 million patients are affected by healthcare-caused infections
15 every year. In the United States, a shocking report suggested that medical errors or adverse events contribute as many as 400,000 deaths per year, making it the third most common cause of death in the country. [1] In response, as much as 76 to 126 billion dollars is spent
20 each year in the United States on medical malpractice lawsuits. [2] These startling statistics seem to suggest that medical providers might not be doing a good job, but there are explanations for them.

🎧 1-30

To be able to grasp the big picture, it is crucial to
25 understand the differences between simple human errors, adverse events, and negligence. First, a simple human error is an unintentional slip that anyone can make. For example, you might have had the experience of pressing the "close" button instead of the "open" button by

rash ／発疹	

frontline ／前線

life threatening ／命に関わる

adverse event ／有害事象

infection ／感染症

denial ／否定

malpractice ／医療過誤、医療ミス

lawsuit ／訴訟

startling ／衝撃的な

statistics ／統計

crucial ／極めて重要な

negligence ／義務を怠ること、過失

unintentional ／故意ではない

slip ／誤り、ミス

mistake while helping someone rushing into an elevator. Anyone can make unintentional mistakes, and medical professionals are no exception. The only way to reduce such errors is to safeguard against them (e.g. by getting

safeguard ／〜を防ぐ

5 rid of the "close" button).

🎧 1-31

An adverse event is a harmful event caused by medicine, but it is not caused by mistakes. For example, having surgery generally carries a 3-to-4 percent risk of infection even if the surgery is performed perfectly. [2] Since human

10 bodies are highly complex, medicine always carries an unpredictable potential for complications. There is no way to reduce the risk of adverse events to zero, since they are by-products of medicine.

by-product ／副産物

🎧 1-32

Lastly, negligence means not giving someone the best

15 care available at the time. Unlike simple human errors or adverse effects, negligence is caused by a wrong decision. For instance, if the best option available for an infection is antibiotic treatment, but no decision is made to use it, this is considered negligence. Prevention of

20 negligence depends on the efforts of individuals, and negligence is often what separates good healthcare providers from the not-so-good.

🎧 1-33

When unfortunate incidents happen in hospitals, whether they are caused by simple human error, an adverse event,

25 or negligence, many people assume that whoever took care of them were the "bad people." But in fact, less than one percent of medical lawsuits in the United States, for instance, are considered to be actual cases of negligence. [2]

Now, which of the three causes above applies to the case

30 of the rash earlier? The answer depends on the situation, and that is exactly why it would not be appropriate to

simply blame the individual. Instead of playing the blame game on an individual level, facility-wide and nationwide interventions need to take place to prevent harm to patients.

blame game ／非難合戦

intervention ／介入

1. Culture of Blame-An Ongoing Burden for Doctors and Patient Safety, International Journal of Environmental Research and Public Health, 2019
2. Negligence, Genuine Error, and Litigation, International Journal of General Medicine, 2013

WPM 550語÷(読むのにかかった時間[秒]÷60) = (　　　　　　　　　　)WPM

Reading Comprehension

下記の英文を読み、本文の内容に合っているものにはT、誤っているものにはFを記入しましょう。

1. One in ten patients in developed countries experience harm caused by errors or adverse events while receiving hospital care. ____

2. An adverse event is a harmful event caused by a wrong decision. ____

3. Negligence is an unintentional slip that anyone can make. ____

4. Medical professionals are exceptions in that they do not make simple human mistakes because they are very careful. ____

5. The risk of infection while undergoing surgery is avoidable if it is performed perfectly. ____

6. Facility-wide and nationwide interventions need to take place to prevent harm to patients. ____

Practice Conversation 1-34

薬局での会話を聞いて、空欄にあてはまる語句を記入しましょう。
答えを確認した後、ペアになって会話を練習しましょう。

Pharmacist: Here's the prescription for your child, ma'am. **Can you confirm your child's name and his date of birth?**

Patient's mother: His name is Jack Williams, [1.   ] on January 1, 2018.

Pharmacist: OK. **Is he allergic to any medications?**

Patient's mother: Not that I know of.

Pharmacist: Here's his prescription.

Patient's mother: Thanks. What is this [2.   ]?

Pharmacist: This is an [3.   ] for his ear [4.   ]. He needs to take it for 10 days.

Patient's mother: Is there anything that I need to watch for?

Pharmacist: The main [5.   ] [   ] of this medication are upset stomach and [6.   ] in some children.

Patient's mother: That doesn't sound good. Is there anything else he can take without the risk of the side effects?

Pharmacist: Unfortunately, any medication carries certain risks. Has he ever had any [7.   ] events before?

Patient's mother: No.

Pharmacist: It may be helpful to take it with food. That would prevent him [8.   ] having an upset stomach. **You can contact us anytime if you have any concerns.**

Patient's mother: OK, thank you for your help.

Useful Expressions 1-35

- **Can you confirm your name and date of birth?**
  (お名前と生年月日の確認をお願いしてもよろしいでしょうか。)

- **Are you allergic to any medications?** (薬アレルギーはありますか。)

- **You can contact us anytime if you have any concerns.**
  (何かご心配なことがあればいつでもご連絡ください。)

Writing Tips

Paraphrasing

あらかじめ読んだり聞いたりした内容を自分の言葉を使って説明することを Paraphrasing（言い換え）と言います。Paraphrasing は、文章の中で資料を引用する場合などに使うライティングの方法です。

【原文例】

This is understandable because medical accidents can be life threatening.

【言い換え例】

This is reasonable since medical errors can be fatal.

このように、文章全体の意味は保ったまま、同義語を使って言い回しを変え、原文とは異なる文章に仕上げることも一つの方法です。同義語が思い浮かばないときには、類語辞典が役に立ちます。

◤Activities

以下のシナリオに沿って、英語で文章を書きましょう。

> **シナリオ:**あなたは、ある病院の安全管理責任者です。最近、抗生物質を投与された患者に全身の発疹と発熱があり、「あのやぶ医者に過失がある」と病院にクレームがありました。調査してみると、過去に薬アレルギーもなく、患者の症状に対して適切に処方されていたことがわかったため、この件は、まれにある抗生物質の副作用による有害事象であるとの結論に至りました。あなたは、有害事象と過失の違いについて患者にわかりやすく説明しなければなりません。

▶有害事象と過失の違いについて、患者にわかるように丁寧な説明を英語で書きましょう。

_____

_____

_____

_____

_____

_____

▶ペアになり、安全管理責任者役と患者役を決め、作文した内容を患者役に説明しましょう。患者役は、説明に対して英語で一言感想を述べましょう。終わったら役を交代しましょう。

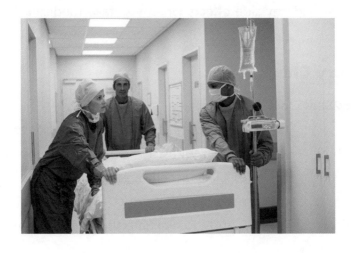

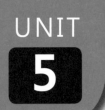

UNIT 5

How Are Drugs Developed?

薬ができるまで

私達が普段飲んでいる薬は、どのように作られているのでしょうか。薬が店頭に並ぶまでには、約10年以上に及ぶ長い道のりがあるのです。その道のりについて順を追って見てみましょう。

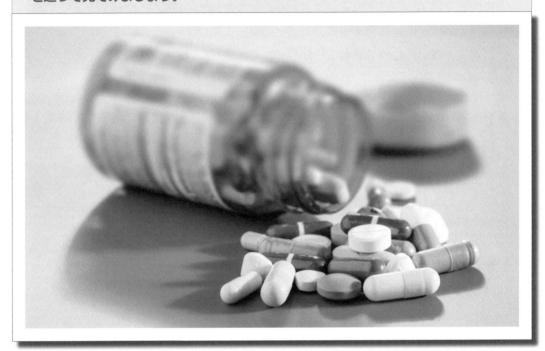

⫸Pre-Reading Questions

ペアになり、以下について話し合いましょう。

Have you ever had any side effects when you take medicines?

⫸Vocabulary Check

次の単語とその定義を結びつけましょう。

1. develop   (a) one of the stages of a process of development
2. clinical study   (b) a formal request for permission to do something
3. phase   (c) to officially accept a plan, proposal
4. approve   (d) to make a new product over a period of time
5. application   (e) any study to evaluate the effects on health outcomes

Reading Tips

Paragraph Reading

長い英文を読むときに、途中で疲れてしまったり、内容を見失ったりすることはありませんか。そんなときは、パラグラフ・リーディングをしてみましょう。英文では、各パラグラフの1文目に最も重要な文が入っていることがほとんどです。その特性を生かして、各パラグラフの最初の1文のみを拾って読んでいくのが、パラグラフ・リーディングです。

下記の英文の全体を読む前に、各パラグラフの1文目に下線を引いて、そこだけ読み通してみましょう。きっと、大まかな内容がつかめて読みやすくなるはずです。

Reading

下記の英文を読みましょう。

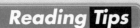 1-36

How long do you think it takes to develop a new drug? In Japan, the usual time span is about nine to 17 years. Also, making a new drug requires a huge amount of money. Each drug costs about 50 billion yen, but only
5 one in 30,000 drugs is successfully developed. Developing a new drug requires several stages. Let's review them one by one.

Early development stage: If a researcher finds a substance that may be useful in curing a disease, it is tried out on
10 animals. At this stage, researchers try to ensure the safety and the efficacy of the drug, and see what toxic effects it shows. At this stage, 466 out of 467 drugs[1] are rejected since they are either too toxic or not very effective.

require ／必要とする	
billion ／ 10 億	
stage ／段階	
one by one ／ 1 つずつ	
substance ／物質	
cure ／治す	
toxic ／毒の	
reject ／拒否する	

If a drug makes it through the early development process, it proceeds to clinical studies.

🎧 1-37

Clinical studies are forms of research that explore whether a medical treatment is safe and effective for
5 humans. In Japan, if the PMDA (Pharmaceuticals and Medical Devices Agency) approves the application of the study, the drug can be tested on people. The clinical studies occur in several phases and only with volunteers who have given their informed consent. All the clinical
10 studies must comply with specific regulations, i.e. GCP (Good Clinical Practice).[2] The following are the three phases.

🎧 1-38

In a Phase 1 study, the drug's safety and toxicity in people are evaluated. Various amounts of the drug are given to
15 a small number of very healthy, young people (usually male) to determine the dose at which toxicity first appears and identify how the compound is absorbed, distributed, metabolized, and excreted. Each volunteer is paid between 10,000 and 100,000 yen. It sounds lucrative,
20 but think very carefully before taking the job, since it may have unexpected effects on your body.

The purpose of a Phase 2 study is twofold: to assess the drug's effect on the disease in question and to calculate the correct dosage. About 100 people who have the
25 target disorder are given different doses of the drug to see whether there are any effects. Even if a drug has proved effective in animal testing, there is no guarantee that these results will be replicated in human beings.

In the Phase 3 study, the drug is tested on more
30 participants who have the target disease. The drug's effectiveness is studied in detail, and any side effects are noted. At this stage, researchers are on the lookout for what these side effects may be and how often they occur, as well as whether factors such as age and sex

process ／過程
proceed to ／～に進む

explore ／見る、調べる

PMDA ／医薬品医療機器総合機構

volunteer ／志願者
informed consent ／説明と同意、同意説明文書

dose ／投与量
compound ／成分
absorb ／吸収する
distribute ／分布する
metabolize ／代謝する
excrete ／排泄する
lucrative ／もうかる
unexpected ／予期しない

participant ／参加者
in detail ／詳細に

make people more susceptible to them.

susceptible ／影響を受
けやすい

🎧 1-39

After the clinical trial, a report is submitted to the PMDA for thorough review. If studies indicate that the drug is effective and safe, a new drug application is filed with
5 the authority. Drug filing documents include a huge amount of data including data from the animal and human tests, intended drug manufacturing procedures, and prescribing information. After approval, the drug finally becomes available for use. Unexpected side effects
10 are continuously monitored even after the release of the drug.

submit ／提出する

authority ／当局

Altogether, it would normally take about 10 years for a drug to go through every stage of testing. But to put the drug development process into perspective, it is
15 important to note that out of 4,000 drugs studied in the laboratory, only around five are studied in human subjects. And out of these drugs, only about 20 percent are approved and prescribed. In a way, every medication is "a miracle drug."

1. 新医薬品の開発成功率（日本製薬工業会）より。1986～1990年の５年間の調査結果
2. GCP：医薬品の臨床試験の実施基準。日米EUの三極で調和された、治験の質を確保するための治験の実施に関する基準のこと。

WPM 589語÷（読むのにかかった時間［秒］÷60）＝（　　　　　　　）WPM

Reading Comprehension

下記の表を、本文の内容を基にして、（　）に適切な日本語を書き入れましょう。

相	薬を投与する対象	目　的	期間
開発初期			
	培養細胞や動物	薬の化学的・物理学的特性を解明し、生物に対する (1.　　　　　　) と (2.　　　　　　) を評価する。	2～ 6.5 年
臨床試験			
第Ⅰ相	健康な人	(3.　　　　　　) を変えながら投与を行い、成分がどのように(4.　　　　　)され、(5.　　　　　)され、代謝、(6.　　　　　) されるかを調べる。	1.5 年

45

第Ⅱ相	治療しようとしている病気にかかっている人、またはかかる可能性がある人最大100人	薬の有効性と使用できる投与量の範囲を調べ、副作用を見つける。	2年
第Ⅲ相	治療しようとしている病気にかかっている人300〜3万人	第Ⅲ相試験では、(7.　　　　　　) の内容と発生頻度、そして発生しやすい年齢、性別などの要素を詳しく調べるとともに、その薬を、すでに発売されている薬やプラセボ（効き目のない偽の薬）と比較検討する。	3.5年
PMDA の審査			
	開発初期と臨床試験からの全ての情報についての審査	薬の (8.　　　　　) と (9.　　　　　　) が立証されたかどうか審査する。	0.5〜1年

▨ Practice Conversation

CD 1-40

クリニックでの会話を聞いて、空欄にあてはまる語句を記入しましょう。
答えを確認した後、ペアになって会話を練習しましょう。

Clinical Research Coordinator (CRC)*: Thank you again for your interest in participating in the clinical [1.　　　] of this new drug. It's nice to finally see you in person, Ms. Suzuki.

Participant: Nice to meet you, too.

CRC: Have you had a chance to read through the informed [2.　　　　　] form that I sent to you last week?

Participant: Yes, I have. I understand that this new drug has already gone through the studies on safety and [3.　　　　　] in people.

CRC: Yes, exactly. We have already finished studying the safe [4.　　　] as well. With the study this time, we would like to see if the drug will actually be [5.　　　　].

Participant: I see. As long as the safety part is taken care of, I would like to try any options we have to feel better. Where do I sign?

CRC: Before you sign this form, did you have any questions about potential [6.　　] [　　　　]?

Participant: No. We already reviewed this part in [7.　　　　] last time.

CRC: OK, then. **Can you please sign here?**

Participant: OK. Here you go.

CRC: Thank you. **Here's your copy.** I'll be working with your doctor to [8.   ] you closely for the next few months. **I'll be contacting you soon.**

Participant: Sounds good.

*clinical research coordinator 治験コーディネーター

Useful Expressions

 1-41

- **Can you please sign here?**（ここに署名をお願いします。）

- **Here's your copy.**（こちらがお控えです。[患者さんのレシートや承諾書など]）

- **I'll be contacting you soon.**（近いうちにご連絡差し上げます。）

Activities

1. 医薬品の開発業界では、多くの略語が使われます。略語は、普段の会話で日常的に飛び交っています。なかでも特によく使われる、治験業界の会社や職種を表す略語の正式名称を英語で書きましょう。また、1～6の空欄に入る単語を表の下の［　］から選び記入しましょう。

略　語	正式名称	日本語	意　味
CRO		開発業務受託機関	[1.]などの治験依頼者に代わり開発業務を行う会社。
SMO		治験施設支援機関	治験を行っている[2.]などの治験実施施設を支援する会社。
CRC		治験コーディネーター	治験実施施設で、担当[3.]の指示のもと治験を円滑に行う為にコーディネートする職種。
CRA		臨床開発モニター	治験依頼者により任命され[4.]を行う職種。治験実施施設を訪問し、治験が予定通りに進行しているのか監査を行う。
MR		医薬情報担当者	主に製薬会社に所属して、[5.]の適正使用に関して、医薬関係者を訪問し、適正使用情報を提供し、情報収集する職種。
SMA		治験事務局担当者	CRCやCRA、治験担当医が治験をスムーズに行えるように、治験に必要な[6.]の作成や管理、各種委員会などの運営支援をする職種。

［　病院　　モニタリング　　書類　　製薬企業　　医師　　医薬品　］

2. 以下のシナリオについて考え、自分の意見を英語で述べましょう。

> **シナリオ：**抗ウイルス薬 A は、新型ウイルスの流行中、海外の複数の医療機関
> で患者に投与され、本格的な臨床試験が始まっていました。ただ、この薬は動物
> 実験で妊娠時の胎児の奇形の発生率を高めることが報告されるなど、副作用の
> 危険もありました。このため投与にあたり必要性を慎重に検討することにしてい
> ます。あなたはこの薬 A を日本の患者に積極的に投与すべきかどうかを決断し、
> 発信する立場にいます。

まず最初に、賛成か反対かを述べます。

賛成 I agree with

反対 I don't agree with / I am opposed to -ing

次に、その理由を述べます。

First of all, / First, / Firstly,（第一に）

Second, / Secondly,（第二に）

Finally, / Lastly,（最後に）

- _____
- _____
- _____

最後に、賛成か反対かの主張を繰り返します。

To sum up, / In summary,   I don't agree with / I am opposed to -ing

---

▶クラスメイトに向けて、あなたの意見をプレゼンテーションしましょう。プレゼンテー
ションを聞いたクラスメイトは、それに対して自分の意見を述べましょう。

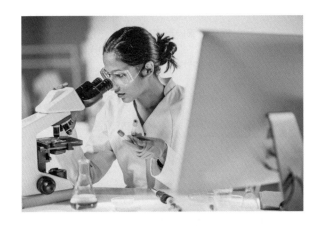

What Comes First when Helping Others

医療従事者も患者？

人の命や健康を守る仕事をする人にとって、まず自分の安全と健康を守ることは、職務をこなす上で最も大切なことである反面、目の前の職務に追われる中で最も忘れがちなことの一つでもあります。医療従事者の健康とそれに関する社会的な課題について見てみましょう。

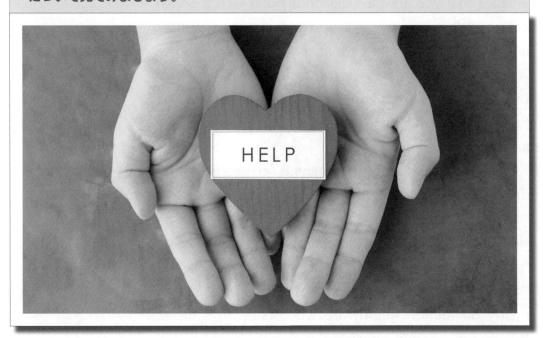

Pre-Reading Questions

ペアになり、以下について話し合いましょう。

What kind of health risks do you think that healthcare workers face at their workplace?

Vocabulary Check

次の単語とその定義を結びつけましょう。

1. pharmacist   **(a)** a condition of being at risk or unprotected
2. exposure   **(b)** a form of energy produced during a nuclear reaction
3. respiratory   **(c)** someone who is an expert on nutrition
4. radiation   **(d)** relating to a process of breathing air in and out
5. nutritionist   **(e)** a person licensed to prepare and dispense drugs

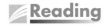

Reading

下記の英文を読みましょう。

 1-42

If you have ever traveled by plane, you may know that every commercial airplane is equipped with oxygen masks stored above your head in case of decompression. Imagine that you are traveling on a plane with a 5-year

5 old boy. What would you do first with the oxygen mask if it dropped down right in front of you? The appropriate action would be to put your own mask on first and help the boy next. Many people may be familiar with the basic rule, "help yourself before you help others," in any

10 lifesaving situation. This rule, however, may not be the case as much as you would imagine for people whose daily role is to save lives, namely healthcare workers.

decompression ／減圧

 1-43

Hospitals and clinics are primarily viewed as places to "receive" care, but at the same time they are places to

15 "give" care. In fact, they are the daily workplaces of nearly 60 million healthcare workers worldwide. [1] Healthcare workers consist of not only doctors and nurses but also all people engaged in actions whose primary aim is to enhance health. They include, but are

20 not limited to, paramedics, dentists, pharmacists, environmental and hygiene health professionals, physiotherapists, nutritionists, laboratory technicians, and assistants of different professions. [2][3] Indeed, healthcare workers account for as much as 12 percent of

25 the total workforce in the world. [3]

paramedic ／救急救命士

hygiene ／衛生

physiotherapist ／理学療法士

laboratory technician ／検査技師

workforce ／労働人口

 1-44

Occupational health is a branch of the medical field that focuses on prevention of health and safety hazards in the workplace. [4] Since healthcare workers are expected to care for others, their own health has been often

occupational health ／労働衛生

hazard ／危険、危害

overlooked by many, including healthcare workers themselves. In recent years, however, the field of occupational health has been increasingly shedding light on healthcare workers themselves as a "patient"
5 population. It has been shown that healthcare workers are more likely to get sick or injured compared to non-healthcare workers. [2][3]

🎧 1-45

The type of health and safety hazard risks for healthcare workers is broad and complex. Some of the major
10 hazards include biological, chemical, physical, ergonomic, and psychosocial hazards. Biological hazards include risks of infection, such as tuberculosis, HIV, hepatitis, and other acute respiratory diseases. Chemical hazards come from exposure to different toxic chemical agents handled in
15 medical settings. Physical hazards include noise, radiation, and slips and falls. Ergonomic hazards are mainly associated with heavy lifting. Psychosocial hazards include shift work, violence, and stress. Across all types of hazards, needle stick injuries, radiation exposure,
20 violence, psychiatric disorders, and suicides are reported to be common in healthcare workers. [1][2]

🎧 1-46

Looking at the long list of hazards, healthcare workers seem well qualified to be high-risk patients, who urgently require more attention and effective intervention on a
25 large scale. Not only do those hazards affect health on an individual level, but unsafe working conditions have also been known to contribute to an acute global shortage of medical staff as well as poor quality of healthcare delivery. [1] Now is the time to come back to
30 the basic rule of lifesaving. Healthcare workers need to be better taken care of, so they can save more lives with their much-needed skills, knowledge, and passion.

---

overlook ／見落とす、目をつぶる

shed light on ／浮き彫りにする

ergonomic ／人間工学の

psychosocial ／心理社会的な

tuberculosis ／結核

hepatitis ／肝炎

needle stick injury ／針刺し損傷

psychiatric ／精神の

qualified ／資格を満たした

intervention ／介入

shortage ／不足

1. Health Worker Occupational Health, World Health Organization, 2020

2. Health Problems in Healthcare Workers: A Review, Journal of Family Medicine and Primary Care, 2019

3. Mapping the Scientific Research on Healthcare Workers' Occupational Health: A Bibliometric and Social Network Analysis, International Journal of Environmental Research and Public Health, 2020.

4. Occupational Health, World Health Organization, 2020.

WPM 510語÷(読むのにかかった時間［秒］÷60) = (　　　　　　　　　)WPM

Reading Comprehension

下記の英文を読み、本文の内容に合っているものにはT、誤っているものにはFを記入しましょう。

1. Doctors and nurses account for as much as 12 percent of the total workforce in the world. ＿＿＿

2. Healthcare workers are more likely to be healthier than the general population. ＿＿＿

3. Occupational health research has been increasingly paying attention to the health and safety of healthcare workers in recent years. ＿＿＿

4. Healthcare workers are exposed to risks of physical hazards, such as noise, radiation, and slips and falls. ＿＿＿

5. An acute global shortage of medical staff may be caused by unsafe working conditions. ＿＿＿

◪Practice Conversation 1-47

企業のオフィスの一室での会話を聞いて、空欄にあてはまる語句を記入しましょう。
答えを確認した後、ペアになって会話を練習しましょう。

Occupational Health Nurse*: **Thank you so much for your time,** Mr. Kumer. Let's review the results of your health checkup* last month, [1.   ] we?

Worker: Sure. Good news? … Or bad news?

Occupational Health Nurse: Please don't worry. It was good overall.

Worker: I'm glad.

Occupational Health Nurse: There was just one thing that I wanted to ask you about. You scored high on the mental health screening. Is there any chance that you may be [2.   ] a lot of stress lately?

Worker: It's hard to admit, but yes. Lately, I've been working way too much. We have a [3.   ] of staff in our IT department.

Occupational Health Nurse: I see.

Worker: I feel so tired, and I have trouble [4.   ]. I also have lower back pain from sitting [5.   ] my desk all day.

Occupational Health Nurse: I think you're [6.   ] for taking a few days off. You can't [7.   ] the importance of good sleep. Would you like me to refer you to a doctor for your sleep issue?

Worker: No, I think I'm OK with taking some rest for now.

Occupational Health Nurse: OK. I also think that using an [8.   ] chair would be helpful for your back pain. **Let me show you how to use it.**

*occupational health nurse 産業保健師 *health checkup 健康診断

◪Useful Expressions 1-48

• **Thank you so much for your time.**（お時間いただきありがとうございます。）

• **Let me show you how to use it.**（使い方をお教えします。）

Writing Tips

Expressing Your Opinion, Part 2

簡単な単語で (S)(V) を組み合わせて自分なりの意見を表現することに少し慣れてきたら、強調したいポイントに次の副詞や形容詞を付け足してみましょう。

I believe that ... → I <u>strongly</u> believe that ... または I <u>truly</u> believe that .....

In my opinion... → In my <u>honest</u> opinion...

これらの表現を使うことで、あなたの意見がより強調されて読み手や聞き手に伝わりやすくなります。ただし、使いすぎるとくどくなってしまうので、一番強調したいポイントに絞って使いましょう。

Activities

以下のシナリオに沿って、あなたの提案を英語で書きましょう。

> **シナリオ：**あなたはある病院の責任者です。最近、世界的に流行している感染症の影響により、外来には沢山の患者が検査を求めて並び、病棟では入院患者も増えています。日を追うごとに、人材や物資の不足が進み、スタッフも疲弊してきています。以下の2種類の危害からできる限り職員を守るために、どのような対策が大切だと考えますか。

1. An example of a biological hazard（生物学的危害の例）：

_____

_____

_____

_____

Your idea :

_____

_____

_____

_____

2. An example of a psychosocial hazard（心理社会的危害の例）:

_____

_____

_____

_____

Your idea :

_____

_____

_____

_____

▶ペアになり、作文したことを共有しましょう。パートナーの発表に対して、英語で一言
感想を述べましょう。

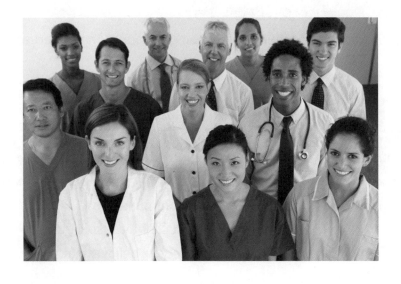

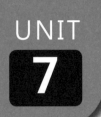

UNIT 7

How to Identify Reliable Health Information

信頼できる健康情報の見分け方

私たちは、新聞や雑誌、インターネットなどで健康についてのさまざまな広告を目にします。中にはいかにも怪しい内容のものもあります。信頼できる医療情報をどのようにして見分けたらよいのか、詳しく見ていきましょう。

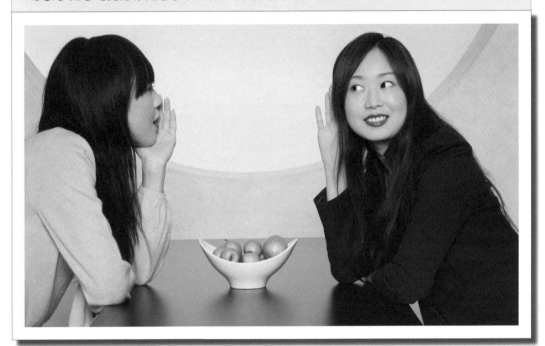

Pre-Reading Questions

ペアになり、以下について話し合いましょう。

Have you ever tried anything after seeing an appealing advertisement?

Vocabulary Check

次の単語とその定義を結びつけましょう。

1. dubious   (a) a strong feeling against one group of people
2. evidence   (b) the person or agency with the power to make decisions
3. authority   (c) informal oral communication
4. bias   (d) not certain and slightly suspicious
5. word-of-mouth   (e) facts that make you believe that something is true

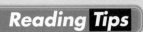

Reading Tips

Paraphrasing

英文でわかりにくい表現に出会ったときは、それを自分にわかる言葉で言い直してみるとわかりやすいです。それは細かいところにこだわらず、そこで何を言いたいのかを考えることができるからです。例えば、

Some ads say," You'll lose 10 kg in weight in one month!" or" This tablet heals any disease." という文章は、「過度に効果をアピールしている広告がある」とまとめてパラフレージング（言い換え）します。

Reading

下記の英文を読みましょう。

🎧 1-49

There is a large amount of health information on the Internet. Some ads say, "You'll lose 10 kg in weight in one month!" or "This tablet heals any disease." These claims are clearly dubious, but in many cases, we do not
5　know how to identify reliable health information.

Why do we consider some information dubious? The reason is that it is not backed up by any evidence. Evidence consists of facts supporting a claim. In the world of medicine, evidence-based medicine (EBM) is
10　regarded as the gold standard. Such evidence comes from the result of many clinical studies. Above all, randomized controlled trials (RCTs) are the most reliable type of clinical trial. The reason why such trials are reliable is that random allocation creates no room for
15　bias. It is tempting for researchers to present data which are desirable for only themselves. Such distortion of

claim ／主張

identify ／見分ける

reliable ／信頼できる

back up ／支持する

gold standard ／金科玉条

RCT ／ランダム化比較試験

allocation ／割り当て

room ／余地

tempting ／誘惑するような

distortion ／歪曲

scientific data is regarded as "unscientific."

 1-50

Data from qualitative studies such as interviews are not so reliable in light of EBM but aren't necessarily useless. Qualitative study data use information gathered from a
5 study that is not based on objective data. Emotions, value of life, and the life history of patients are not based on numbers or facts, but are very important when medical professionals provide patients with tailor-made treatments. This undoubtedly contributes to improving
10 patients' quality of life (QOL). Narrative-based medicine (NBM), which values a patient's story, is a newly developed field of medicine.

Evidence drawn from the opinion of authorities is the least reliable, and word-of-mouth information is not even
15 considered to be evidence. An expert opinion must not be confused with personal opinion. Personal opinion is not acceptable as evidence. Even if ads are attractive and well-made and the user sounds persuasive, there is no scientific value in this information. Then how can we
20 identify reliable health information? The following are some tips that may help you do so:

 1-51

1. Always research reliable sources.
Reliable sources include government websites, government-related organizations, large academic
25 associations, and hospitals.

2. Think 5W1H for the information.
Consider not only what is provided as information, but also confirm when the data were gathered. Nobody wants to rely on old information. If the information is not
30 acquired from reliable sources where there is appropriate facility to get correct data, the information might be dubious. Also, think about whether there is someone who will benefit as a result of the health information (the reason why someone claims it). Is this spokesperson fair

qualitative study ／質的研究
objective ／客観的な

narrative ／語り

source ／(情報)源

benefit ／利益を得る

and honest? Lastly, check how the information was provided. Exaggerated information may cause misunderstanding. See information from various angles.

3. Ask health professionals if your understanding is
5   correct.

health professional ／医療従事者

There might be an information source that health professionals take for granted but is unfamiliar to the general public. The expert might have a special network. Consulting an expert allows us to think about facts from
10 various perspectives. Experts can answer your questions.

take for granted ／当然と思う

perspective ／見地

🎧 1-52

Now you have learned how to identify reliable health information. This ability is called health literacy. The World Health Organization defines health literacy as the social skills that determine the ability of individuals to
15 understand and use information. Good health literacy is crucial for our daily lives, as it allows us to maintain good health.

WPM 539語÷（読むのにかかった時間［秒］÷60）＝（   ）WPM

Reading Comprehension

下記の表は、信頼できる健康情報を見分ける方法をまとめたものです。（　）内に適切な日本語を書き入れましょう。

	タイトル	方　　法
1	信頼できる情報源	(1.)、(2.)、(3.) や病院などの信頼できる情報源から、常に情報を探すようにする。
2	情報の5W1Hを考える	What：(4.) として何が提供されているか。 When：そのデータが得られた (5.)。 Where：正確なデータを得るために (6.) な施設なのか。 Who：その健康情報によって誰かが (7.) をしていないか。 Why：なぜその情報が (8.) されているのか。 How：(9.) その情報が提供されているか。誇張はないか。
3	医療者に尋ねる	自分の考えがそれで正しいか医療者に尋ねてみる。専門家であれば、事実を (10.) な (11.) から検討できる。

▰ Practice Conversation

 1-53

トラベルクリニックでの会話を聞いて、空欄にあてはまる語句を記入しましょう。
答えを確認した後、ペアになって会話を練習しましょう。

Nurse: Thank you for filling out the form, Mr. Yamada. So, you're going to South America?

Patient: Yes, my roommate told me that I need to get a lot of vaccinations before I leave.

Nurse: **It depends**. All vaccines have [1.   ] and [2.   ], and I would like to ask you some questions first before discussing further options with the doctor.

Patient: Oh, OK. I guess I was being too nervous about what he told me.

Nurse: Can I ask what you'll be doing in South America?

Patient: I'll be backpacking. I've [3.   ] that there's some kind of scary virus going around. Do I need to get a vaccine for that?

Nurse: We'll see. Sometimes, [4.   ] information can be [5.   ]. **Do you mind if I show you** some websites we use?

Patient: Sure.

Nurse: These are some of the [6.   ] sources that we refer to. All the recommendations here are [7.   ] up by evidence.

Patient: Oh, I see. I guess I don't need to have a lot of vaccines after all. This is helpful.

Nurse: It's also important to check the websites of the local [8.   ] and embassies* while you're there.

Patient: OK, thanks for the information.

*embassy 大使館

▰ Useful Expressions

 1-54

- **It depends.** (ケースバイケースです。)

- **Do you mind if I show you.......?**
  (〜[ウェブサイト、本、資料など]をお見せしましょうか。)

Activities

信用できない健康情報は、世の中にあふれています。今までに出会った怪しげな広告を思い出して、どの点が疑わしかったのか、どう疑わしかったのか振り返ってみましょう。下記の空欄に英語で記入しましょう。

怪しげな広告（どんな広告？）	どの点が疑わしかったのか？	どう疑わしかったのか？

▶作成した表を基に、信頼できる医療情報を得るためには普段からどのように考え、行動したらよいか、自分の考えを英語で書きましょう。

_____

_____

_____

_____

_____

_____

▶以上のことを英語でまとめて作文し、グループで発表しましょう。クラスメイトが発表したら、それに対して英語で一言意見を言いましょう。

_____

_____

_____

_____

_____

_____

_____

_____

_____

_____

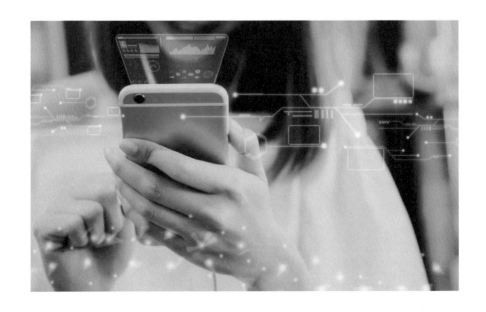

What Is "Upstream" Thinking?

「上流」思考とは？

「公衆衛生」と聞いて何を思い浮かべますか。多くの人はぼんやりとしたイメージしかありませんが、地域規模、さらには地球規模の大きな医療課題に取り組む上でとても重要な分野です。公衆衛生の概念を学ぶ上でよく使われる例え話に、どんな教訓が隠されているのか見てみましょう。

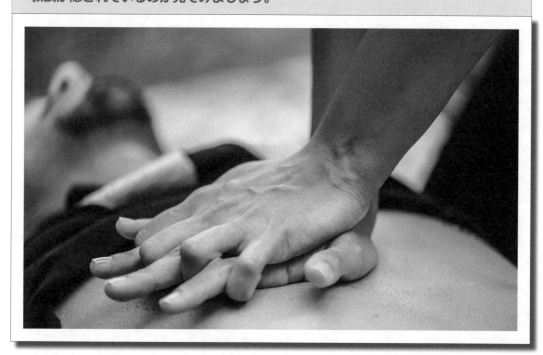

Pre-Reading Questions

ペアになり、以下について話し合いましょう。

What comes to mind when you think about the term "public health"?

Vocabulary Check

次の単語とその定義を結びつけましょう。

1. victim　　　　　　**(a)** very tired

2. artery　　　　　　**(b)** to try to find out the facts about something

3. exhausted　　　　**(c)** a vessel that carries oxygen-rich blood

4. investigate　　　　**(d)** a way of thinking about something

5. perspective　　　　**(e)** someone who has been harmed or injured

⬛ Reading

下記の英文を読みましょう。

🎧 2-01

Once upon a time, there was a small village by a big river at the foot of majestic mountains. This small village was known for a mysterious phenomenon. The villagers found drowning people coming down the river every

5 single day. The villagers were kept extremely busy finding victims and saving their lives in the river downstream. Even though they tried their best, they eventually felt exhausted as the task seemed endless. Looking at the weary villagers one day, a little girl pointed to the

10 mountains and asked a very simple question, "What's happening upstream anyway?" This question opened up a whole new perspective in how to approach the problem. This is one of the parables taught when learning the concept of public health. What kind of

15 lesson do you think is hidden in this story?

phenomenon ／現象

upstream ／上流

parable ／例え話
public health ／公衆衛生学

🎧 2-02

The field of public health aims to answer the same question as the little girl when dealing with a big problem affecting many people. Public health is defined as "the art and science of preventing disease, prolonging

20 life, and promoting health through the organized efforts of society." Public health focuses on the cause of the problem and finding a way to provide conditions under which the health and well-being of people as a whole will be improved. (1)

effort ／努力、取り組み

well-being ／健康で安心なこと、福利、幸福

🎧 2-03

25 The world is facing a pandemic of chronic diseases. Ischemic heart disease and stroke are accountable for nearly 30 percent of all deaths in the world. These chronic conditions have been the biggest causes of death globally for more than 15 years. Ischemic heart

pandemic ／世界に流行している
chronic ／慢性の
ischemic heart disease ／虚血性心疾患
stroke ／脳卒中

disease in particular continues to be the top killer, responsible for nearly 10 million deaths per year. [2] Many cases of ischemic heart disease are caused by a buildup of plaque in the main arteries supplying oxygen to the
5 heart muscle. When the blood cannot pass through the narrowed arteries freely, the heart cannot receive enough oxygen to carry out its functions properly. This condition is experienced as a heart attack. [3]

plaque ／プラーク

heart attack ／心臓発作

🎵 2-04

Knowing that heart attack is taking the lives of so many
10 people worldwide, what would you do to save them? Would you spend all of your time training as many people as possible in CPR? Would you spend all the resources to install AEDs in every corner of the city? They are certainly good things to do. Yet, if so many victims of
15 heart attacks in millions keep "coming down the river," you need to ask, "What's happening upstream anyway?" In other words, you have to dig deeper to answer the critical question, "Why are they here in the first place?"

CPR ／心肺機能蘇生
AED ／自動体外式除細動器

🎵 2-05

After all, everybody seems to know that healthy diet and
20 exercise are important in reducing the risk of ischemic heart disease. Why, then, do so many people still suffer from it? You may find some answers in the socioeconomic context of people, such as living conditions, income, and culture. You may want to study epidemiology, which is a
25 study of cause and effect. You may want to refer to many other areas of study such as social science, behavioral science, and environmental science, for example. Becoming an "upstream" thinker and an effective life saver requires a broad perspective across many different
30 disciplines.

socioeconomic ／社会経済的な
context ／背景
epidemiology ／疫学
cause and effect ／因果、原因と結果

discipline ／分野、学科、領域

🎵 2-06

Instead of trying to help as many drowning people as possible, people in the village needed to find a way to prevent people from drowning in the first place. They went up into the mountains and investigated what was causing the problem upstream. They solved the problem by constructing a durable bridge over the spot in the river where people used to jump from one slippery rock to another, trying to get to the other side. Thanks to their hard work, people can now cross the river safely without getting carried away by the strong current.

1. Public Health Services, World Health Organization Europe, 2020
2. The Top 10 Causes of Death, World Health Organization, 2018
3. Ischemic Heart Disease: An Update, Seminars in Nuclear Medicine, 2020

WPM 625語÷(読むのにかかった時間[秒]÷60) = (　　　　　　　　)WPM

Reading Comprehension

下記の表は、本文の内容をまとめたものです。(　)に入る適切な英単語を語群から選び記入しましょう。

	Problem	"Downstream" Thinking	"Upstream" Thinking
Village	So many drowning people keep coming down the river every day.	Finding and saving the (1.　　　　　) as they come until villagers get (2.　　　　　).	Investigating what is happening up in the (5.　　　　　). (6.　　　　　) a durable bridge so people do not drown in the first place.
Public Health	Ischemic heart disease is killing nearly 10 million people per year.	(3.　　　　　) as many people as possible on how to do CPR until resources run out. (4.　　　　　) as many AEDs as possible throughout the city until resources run out.	Investigating the socioeconomic (7.　　　　　) of people suffering from the disease to find the (8.　　　　　). Collaborating with experts in (9.　　　　　), social science, behavioral science, and environmental science.

語　　群
epidemiology / saving / context / burden / constructing mountains / downstream / removing / training / recovered / exhausted villagers / victims / cause / effect / river / installing

Practice Conversation

 2-07

病室での会話を聞いて、空欄にあてはまる語句を記入しましょう。
答えを確認した後、ペアになって会話を練習しましょう。

Nutritionist: **May I come in?**

Patient: Yes, please do.

Nutritionist: Hi, Mr. Kim. I'm Kay, your nutritionist. How are you feeling today?

Patient: I'm feeling so much better after the [1.　　　　　]. I still can't believe that I had a [2.　　　] attack. I never want to experience that again.

Nutritionist: That must have been so scary.

Patient: Oh, it was terrifying. I was so lucky that my boss knew how to do [3.　　　], and my workplace had an [4.　　　].

Nutritionist: Your doctor has told me to talk to you before you go home. **Would it be OK if I ask you some questions?**

Patient: Sure.

Nutritionist: As you know, the heart attack was caused by a [5.　　　　　] condition that can be improved by [6.　　　] and exercise.

Patient: Yes, I know. It's been hard for me to eat healthily because I've always [7.　　　] so busy.

Nutritionist: I understand. Eating healthily sounds simple, but it's hard for many people.

Patient: I know what to do, but it's hard to actually do it. I don't know where to start.

Nutritionist: Right, that's exactly why I would like to ask you about your lifestyle first. It will be a collaborative [8.　　　] between you and me as well as your family.

Patient: I'm ready to do anything to prevent another heart attack.

Useful Expressions

 2-08

- **May I come in?** （入ってもよろしいですか。）

- **Would it be OK if I ask you some questions?**
  （いくつか質問をさせていただいてもよろしいですか。）

Expressing Your Opinion, Part 3

他人の提案や意見に対して、自分の感想や意見を述べることは、ディスカッションやライティングにおいて必要ですが、慣れていないと難しいものです。以下は相手の意見に対して肯定的・否定的な感想を述べる際に便利な表現です。

【肯定的な例】

I agree with you that..., I have come to the same conclusion that..., I hold the same opinion that..., I think you're right about...

【否定的な例】

I don't necessarily agree with you that..., I have a different view on..., I disagree that...

Activities

すでに病気を患っている人を助けることも、病気を未然に防ぐことも、医療ではどちらのアプローチも大切ですが、地域や国など大きな規模の問題に取り組む際には公衆衛生の「上流」思考が力を発揮します。以下のシナリオに沿って、あなたの提案を英語で述べましょう。

> **シナリオ:**あなたは、ある自治体の保健課の職員です。この市では例年、心臓発作で亡くなったり後遺症を残す高齢者の数が全国平均を大きく上回り、市長は何かいいアイディアはないかと模索しています。あなたは職場の会議で、現状を改善するために、素晴らしい提案を発表します。

State the problem (現在の問題を述べましょう)

_____

_____

_____

State your opinion (あなたの提案を述べましょう)

_____

_____

_____

▼

Support your opinion (その提案が素晴らしい理由を述べましょう)

● _____

● _____

● _____

▼

Restate your opinion (あなたの提案、結論を再度述べましょう)

_____

_____

_____

▶クラスメイトを市長と市の職員と想定して、あなたの提案を発表しましょう。発表を聞いたクラスメイトは、提案に対して Writing Tips を参考に一言自分の感想を英語で述べましょう。

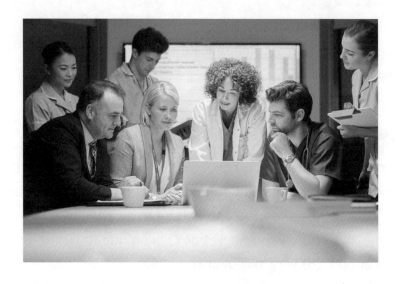

UNIT 9

Actions Speak Louder than Words

非言語コミュニケーションの力

海外からの旅行者や居住者が増える中、未来の医療従事者が、世界の共通語である英語を習得することの重要性は高まっています。医療英語を初めて学ぶ際に気を取られがちなのは数々の難しい専門用語ですが、実際の現場では専門用語や暗記したフレーズを使いこなすことよりもまず重要なことがあります。言葉に頼らないコミュニケーションについて見てみましょう。

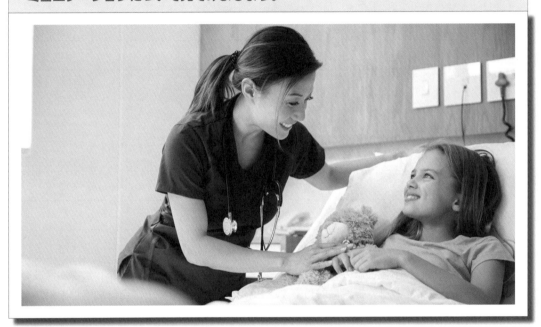

Pre-Reading Questions

ペアになり、以下について話し合いましょう。

What are some ways to communicate with people if you are not familiar with their language ?

Vocabulary Check

次の単語とその定義を結びつけましょう。

1. admit	**(a)**	the ability to understand how someone feels
2. proficient	**(b)**	a tendency to behave in a certain way
3. empathy	**(c)**	a wrong belief or opinion due to lack of understanding
4. misconception	**(d)**	very skillful at something
5. disposition	**(e)**	to take someone into hospital for medical care

Reading Tips

Grasping the Gist

長文を読み進めてみたものの、途中で何の話かわからなくなり、読むのを諦めたくなることはありませんか。いきなり目を通す代わりに、ちょっとした事前準備を習慣にすることで、そんな経験を減らすことができます。具体的には①タイトルの意味を考えてみること、②見出しの文からどのような内容かを予想してみること、③文章中のわからない語の意味を調べておくことを事前に行います。専門書や論文などの難解な文章ほど、これらの作業が助けになります。

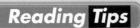

Reading

下記の英文を読みましょう。

2-09

Have you ever gotten sick while traveling in a foreign country? Try to imagine the situation. In pain and discomfort, you finally manage to find a local clinic accepting walk-ins. You are surrounded by people
5 speaking in an unfamiliar language. You are anxiously sitting in a waiting room alone, looking at other patients coming in and out. You cannot see what is going on behind the door. Sick and scared, you cannot help but wonder, "What are they going to do to me?"

10 With Japan hosting nearly 32 million inbound travelers a year, medical personnel proficient in assisting foreign patients are in greater demand than ever. [1] It is reported that about 80 percent of medical facilities in Japan have admitted foreign patients, and nearly 6 percent of those
15 facilities see more than 1,000 foreign patients a year. [2]

discomfort ／不快感、不快症状

walk-in ／予約なしの、飛び込みの

Although those foreign patients consist of travelers and temporary residents of many different native tongues, English remains the most common language of choice when receiving medical care.[2] The importance of learning English as future medical professionals has been increasingly emphasized for a good reason. Overcoming the language barrier, however, is just one aspect of taking care of foreign patients in reality.

aspect ／側面

🎧 2-10

What patients look for, much more so when dealing with an unexpected problem in a foreign country, is the sense of reassurance that they are in "good hands." This sense of reassurance comes from the rapport between medical staff and patients. Rapport refers to a mutual relationship based on agreement, empathy, and understanding. [3] Having rapport is the foundation of good communication. In fact, without first establishing rapport, the knowledge of "what to say" to patients becomes close to useless as it is easily perceived as ingenuine or inappropriate. [4] This is why simply learning supposedly helpful phrases would not be enough in real situations.

reassurance ／安心感

rapport ／ラポール、感情的な親密さ

mutual ／相互の、共通の

ingenuine ／不誠実な

inappropriate ／不適切な

supposedly ／建前では、恐らくは

🎧 2-11

Building rapport requires people to feel that they have something in common, such as ethnic background, gender, social status, age, clothing, hobbies, and so on. [4] Can you imagine how challenging it would be to build rapport with foreign travelers in a clinical setting? On top of the obvious language and cultural barriers, they are likely to be anxious and in pain or discomfort. They may also be under stress due to time constraints as a trip to a hospital is never on their itinerary. Is there anything one can do to establish rapport in a stressful situation, with limited time and lack of common cultural attributes?

constraint ／制約

itinerary ／旅程

attribute ／特質、特性

🎧 2-12

One domain of commonality that anyone can use even in such challenging situations is behavior. There is a

commonality ／（性質などを）共有していること

common misconception among medical professionals that they are to remain "professional," in other words, to stay calm and soft-spoken, no matter how a patient is acting. Although it may seem counter-intuitive, matching

5 the patient's behavior, disposition, and rhythm at the initial encounter has been shown to be the fastest, simplest, and the most effective way to establish rapport. [4]

counter-intuitive ／直感に反した

encounter ／出会い、接触

🎧 2-13

For example, if a patient is acting very anxious, breathing rapidly, and raising his or her voice, a medical professional

10 can match such behavior for a few seconds as a way of acknowledging this emotional state. This act creates an instant bond, in which a medical professional can quickly calm the patient by demonstrating slower breathing and a lower voice in turn. Once this synchronization happens,

15 which could be a matter of a few seconds, the communication following will be much smoother.[4]

synchronization ／同期すること

However intimidating it may seem to assist foreign patients in English, everyone deserves to be comforted with the best effort possible. Instead of worrying about

20 what you say, remember that in the absence of apparent commonality, actions count more than words. Once you have succeeded in establishing rapport, you have already unlocked the key to better, genuine communication that patients will appreciate.

intimidating ／怯えさせるような

genuine ／心からの

appreciate ／よく理解する、感謝する

1. 訪日外客統計,日本政府観光局, 2019
2. 医療機関における外国人旅行者及び在留外国人受入れ体制等の実態調査, 厚生労働省, 2017
3. Rapport, Merriam-Webster Dictionary, 2020
4. A Better Patient Experience through Better Communication, Journal of Radiology Nursing, 2013

WPM 627語÷（読むのにかかった時間［秒］÷60）＝（　　　　　　　　）WPM

Reading Comprehension

下記の英文を読み、本文の内容に合っているものにはT、誤っているものにはFを記入しましょう。

1. Travelers to Japan consist mostly of native English speakers. ____

2. Using supposedly helpful phrases in English may be perceived as inappropriate or ingenuine without first establishing rapport. ____

3. Building rapport requires that people feel that they have something in common. ____

4. Being proficient in the language that the patient is familiar with is the most important aspect of building rapport. ____

5. One of the reasons that foreign travelers are likely to be under stress in a medical setting is that visiting a hospital is something unexpected. ____

6. The best way for medical professionals to calm patients down is to stay calm and soft-spoken at all times. ____

Practice Conversation

CD 2-14

病院の廊下での会話を聞いて、空欄にあてはまる語句を記入しましょう。
答えを確認した後、ペアになって会話を練習しましょう。

Patient: Excuse me. I'm not sure where I'm supposed to go. Can you help me?

Staff: Of course. **Is this your first visit to our hospital?**

Patient: Yes. Actually, I'm traveling in Japan for the first time.

Staff: I'm so sorry that you got sick [1. ____] traveling. It must be [2. ____] to visit a hospital overseas. **What seems to be the problem?**

Patient: I feel really sick [3. ____] my stomach. I think I have a fever as well.

Staff: I see. Our emergency department* is accepting [4. ____] anytime. I can show you where it is.

Patient: I'm relieved to hear that. This was totally [5. ____], and I didn't even know if any place [6. ____] be open in the evening.

Staff: By the way, would you be more comfortable talking to a doctor in a language other [7. ____] English?

Patient: Yes, Mandarin is my native [8.   ].

Staff: Great. We have a translator available.

Patient: **I really appreciate your help.**

*emergency department 救急外来

Useful Expressions 2-15

• **Is this your first visit to our hospital?**（この病院は初めてですか。）

• **What seems to be the problem?**（どうされましたか。）

• **I really appreciate your help.**（本当にありがとうございます。）

Activities

非言語コミュニケーションには、お辞儀、握手、相づち、視線、手の合図、顔の表情、服装、姿勢など、さまざまな動作や行動が含まれます。ペアまたはグループで、興味のある国を選び、その国の非言語コミュニケーション (non-verbal communication) について調べ、動作とその意味の例を 2 つ下の表に英語でまとめましょう。

選んだ国

	動作／行動	意　味
例 1		
例 2		

▶調べたことを下に英語でまとめ、クラスで発表しましょう。

In our group, we looked at some forms of non-verbal communication in
_____ （国名）.

We would like to share a few examples and their meanings.

The first example is

_____

_____

_____

_____

_____

The second example is

_____

_____

_____

_____

_____

Thank you for listening. Do you have any questions?

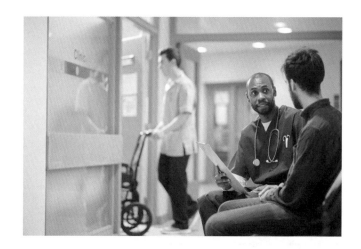

UNIT 10

Genetic Counseling as an Emerging Field

新たな分野、遺伝カウンセリング

遺伝カウンセリングという言葉を知っていますか？ 1996 年 7 月にクローン技術から生まれた世界初の羊のドリーの誕生は、世界中を驚かせました。その結果として、遺伝子の影響力や遺伝性の病気に対して高い関心を持つ人も増えました。しかし、遺伝カウンセリングやカウンセリングを行う遺伝カウンセラーについては、まだ広くは知られていません。

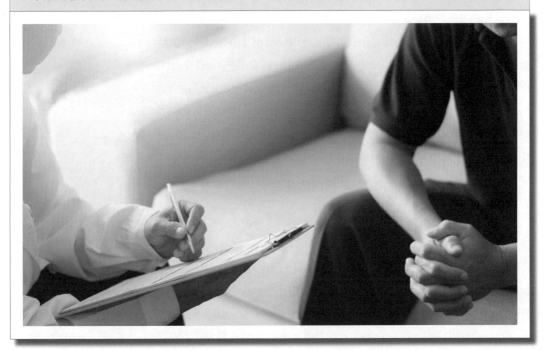

Pre-Reading Questions

ペアになり、以下について話し合いましょう。

Tell your partner everything you can think of about genes.

Vocabulary Check

次の単語とその定義を結びつけましょう。

1. hereditary   **(a)** a state of carrying babies inside one's body
2. family tree   **(b)** a chart that shows all the people in a family
3. pregnancy   **(c)** something that a person has had from birth
4. abortion   **(d)** passing, naturally from parent to children
5. congenital   **(e)** an intentional ending of a pregnancy

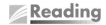

下記の英文を読みましょう。

🎧 **2-16**

Do you know what a genetic counselor is? As research progresses, the subject of human genes has received extensive coverage in newspapers, television, and other media. One milestone was reached in July 1996, when
5 the world heard the amazing news that a sheep named Dolly had become the first such animal to be born using cloning technology. And in 2013, the world learned that superstar Hollywood actress Angelina Jolie had both breasts removed because of the risk of hereditary breast
10 cancer. These and other stories sparked widespread curiosity among the general public in the subject of genetic influences and hereditary diseases. Despite this interest, the activities of genetic counselors are not widely known.

milestone ／（歴史など における）画期的な出来 事

🎧 **2-17**

15 If people have questions about genetics, it is the task of a genetic counselor to provide them with accurate medical information based on scientific evidence. When thinking about genetic problems, patients should review their own illnesses as well as their family's. They must
20 also consider them when making decisions such as whether or not to have a child. In such cases, it is the job of the genetic counselor to provide support not only in medical matters but also for associated psychological and social aspects.

scientific evidence ／ 科学的根拠

psychological ／心理的 な

25 To be certified as a genetic counselor, you naturally need to be familiar with the most up-to-date developments in genetic medicine. In addition, you need to be well-versed in professional counseling, aware of ethical and legal issues, and skilled in teamwork. Certified genetic
30 counselors are accredited as specialists in genetic

certified ／認定を受け た

well-versed ／精通して

ethical ／倫理的な

accredited ／認定された

medicine by a relevant professional body. A clinical genetic specialist must be a qualified doctor, but a genetic counselor does not necessarily have to be a medical professional. As long as you have been educated

5 at a specialized institution, you can work in the medical field even with no medical qualifications.

🎧 2-18

First and foremost, genetic counselors explain to people how genes and genetic counseling works. After that, they gather information about a patient's family and draw up

10 a family tree. In the case of a hereditary disease such as cancer, they will ask if there are any relatives who had the same disease. For those who decide to undergo a genetic test, the counselors will use the results to explain the details and answer questions.

first and foremost ／
何よりもまず

15 Patients who opt to receive genetic counseling may have various motives. They may be worried about a baby having abnormalities during pregnancy or whether genes that caused disease in their parents will also affect them. Your genetic information is vital personal information

20 that remains constant throughout your life. And because you share this information with family members, your own genetic tests may reveal the possibility of the same disease in a blood relative. Genetic counselors must be able to offer psychological and emotional support to

25 patients if they learn bad news.

opt to ／〜することを
選ぶ
motive ／動機

abnormality ／異常

As a general rule, patients must cover the costs of genetic counseling out of their own pocket, and each facility sets its own prices. In some cases, however, insurance may cover the costs.

🎧 2-19

30 More than 4,000 genetic counselors are already active in the United States, where genetic medicine is becoming well established. However, the number of certified genetic counselors in Japan is very small, with just 267

certified practitioners as of April 2020. The salary and conditions of certified genetic counselors vary depending on the hospital or company where they work. However, with demand for their services high, the profession is
5　attracting a lot of attention not only from hospitals and other medical institutions but also from the pharmaceutical, healthcare, and diet industries.

CD 2-20

But there are still legal and ethical issues to be solved. From a legal point of view, some people argue that having
10　direct contact with patients and conducting counseling could constitute a "series of medical practices," which may put genetic counselors in violation of the Medical Act.

series of medical practices ／一連の医療行為

violate ／違反する

Ethical issues include prenatal diagnosis, which could
15　lead to selective abortion. This raises the ethical problem of whether it is correct to choose not to give birth to a baby with congenital disabilities. It is difficult for genetic counselors alone to solve such problems; the response must come from large organizational systems such as
20　genetic clinics attached to university hospitals.

prenatal diagnosis ／出生前診断

selective abortion ／選択的流産

congenital disability ／先天性障害

Legal and ethical problems such as these are currently obstacles to the progress of genetic counseling, and the future development of the field depends on coming up with solutions.

WPM 723語÷(読むのにかかった時間[秒]÷60) = (　　　　　　　　　)WPM

◢Reading Comprehension

下記の表は本文の内容をまとめたものです。(　)に入る英単語を書き入れましょう。

What is genetic counseling?	If people have questions related to genetics, a genetic counseling helps them understand accurate medical information based on (1.　　　　　) (2.　　　　　).

Why is it needed?	An increasing number of people are becoming interested in genetic influence and (3.) (4.). They may worry about a baby's abnormalities during pregnancy, and about whether they have inherited their parents' disease genes.
What does a genetic counselor do?	A genetic counselor provides support not only in medical matters but also with associated (5.) and (6.) aspects.
How can I get certified as a genetic counselor?	To be certified as a genetic counselor, you need up-to-date knowledge of (7.) medicine, professional (8.) techniques, awareness of (9.) (10.) (11.) issues, and skill in (12.).
How is genetic counseling conducted?	Genetic counselors first provide general knowledge about genes and genetic counseling. After that, they gather information about the patient's (13.) while making a (14.) (15.).
Why is it difficult to conduct genetic counseling?	One legal problem is that contacting a patient directly and conducting counseling could constitute a "series of medical practices" and may violate the (16.) (17.). Ethical issues include (18.) (19.), which allows for (20.) (21.).

▰ Practice Conversation

 2-21

産婦人科での会話を聞いて、空欄にあてはまる語句を記入しましょう。
答えを確認した後、ペアになって会話を練習しましょう。

Patient: (Knocking) Come in.

Doctor: Hi. Nice to see you again, Ms. Santos, and **congratulations on** your [1.   ].

Patient: Thank you, doctor. We're so excited.

Doctor: Great. First, I would like to review your medical history*, and we'll do some examinations later.

Patient: I'm ready.

Doctor: On our form, I see that you answered "yes" [2.] the optional* genetic tests for [3.   ] diseases.

Patient: Yes, my sister has a history of pregnancy with [4.   ] abnormalities. She had an [5.   ], unfortunately. That's why we are interested in [6.   ] the tests done.

Doctor: I see. If you're interested, **I would like to introduce you to** our genetic counselor, Ms. Kato, at our next appointment.

Patient: What does a genetic counselor do?

Doctor: A genetic counselor is someone [7.   ] to explain about genetic tests and answer your questions.

Patient: That sounds great. To be honest, I'm so scared about the test results. It would be nice to have someone I can talk to.

Doctor: Exactly. Ms. Kato will work closely with me and will give you [8.   ] and social support if you need. **Would you like to make an appointment with** her?

Patient: Sure. Thank you.

---

*medical history 病歴　*optional 任意の

Useful Expressions 2-22

- **Congratulations on ....** （～[事]おめでとうございます。）

- **I would like to introduce you to......** （～[人]を紹介させていただきます。）

- **Would you like to make an appointment with .....?**
  （～[人]とのご予約をとりましょうか。）

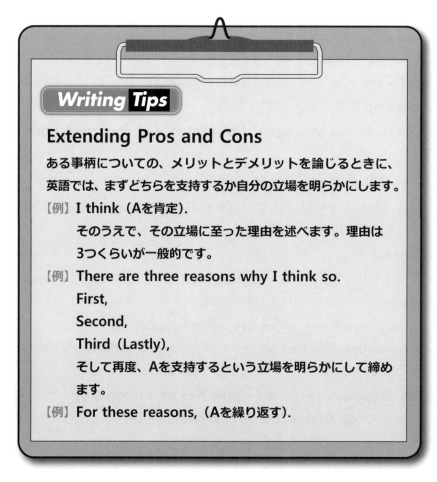

Writing Tips

Extending Pros and Cons

ある事柄についての、メリットとデメリットを論じるときに、英語では、まずどちらを支持するか自分の立場を明らかにします。

【例】 I think (Aを肯定).

そのうえで、その立場に至った理由を述べます。理由は3つくらいが一般的です。

【例】 There are three reasons why I think so.

First,

Second,

Third (Lastly),

そして再度、Aを支持するという立場を明らかにして締めます。

【例】 For these reasons, (Aを繰り返す).

Activities

遺伝カウンセリングの是非について、英語で述べましょう。

Question What do you think are the pros and cons of genetic counseling?

Discuss answers to the question with your partner and write them in the table below.
（問題について、パートナーと話し合い、自分の意見を英語で書きましょう。）

Pros	• • • • •
Cons	• • • • •

After discussing with your partner, share your answers with your classmates.

（パートナーと話し合った後、自分の意見をクラスメイトに英語で発表しましょう。）

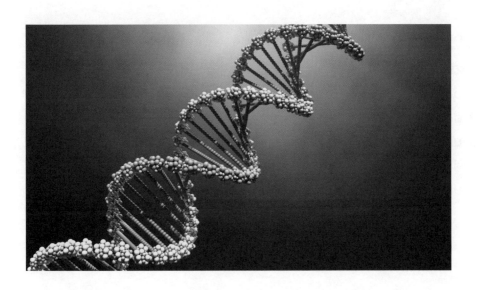

Can Medical Tourism Be a White Knight?

医療ツーリズムは救世主になれるか？

現在、日本の病院の多くは財政上の困難に直面しています。2017年に政府がまとめた報告書によると、公立病院の約6割が赤字経営です。病院は、経営上の活路として、自国で受けられない医療を受けに他国へ行く自由診療の医療ツーリズムに注目するようになりました。医療ツーリズムは、医療経営を救う白馬の王子様になることはできるのでしょうか。

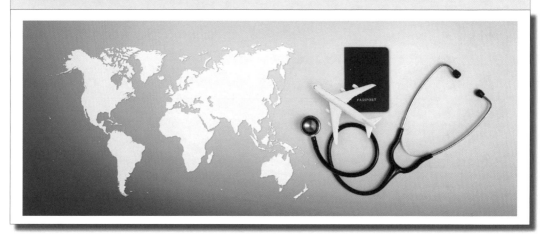

Pre-Reading Questions

ペアになり、以下について話し合いましょう。

What do you think about visiting a hospital abroad?

Vocabulary Check

次の単語とその定義を結びつけましょう。

1. postpone   (a) to ask for something forcefully
2. domestic   (b) not officially accepted
3. unapproved   (c) to delay an event
4. demand   (d) not able to be used or get
5. unavailable   (e) a person's own country

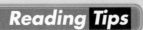

Using Signal Words

文脈の方向転換に使われる signal words を、change-of-direction signals または contrasts といい、although, despite, instead of, even though, nevertheless, on the other hand などが含まれます。例えば、著者が言いたいことに対して否定的な文脈を、肯定的な文脈へと方向転換するときに用いられます。

【例文】

People now desire tailored care chosen from as many options as possible. (ここまでは肯定的)(ここからは否定的) Healthcare providers, on the other hand, may be more careful.

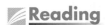

下記の英文を読みましょう。

Currently, many hospitals in Japan are facing financial difficulties. According to a report by the government in December 2017, 60 percent of public hospitals are experiencing such problems. Now hospitals are focusing
5 on a new way to manage their finances: medical tourism.

Medical tourism refers to the practice of going abroad to receive medical care that is unavailable in your home country. This ranges from advanced forms of medical care such as cancer treatment to cosmetic surgery. As of
10 2020, medical tourism is being positioned as a new growth strategy in Japan. Many hospital managers believe that "medical tourists" are willing to pay high prices in exchange for premium health care. The field is drawing attention as a new way to bolster domestic

medical tourism ／医療ツーリズム

cosmetic surgery ／美容整形手術

as of ／～の時点で

growth strategy ／成長戦略

demand as Japan's population continues to decline. In fact, some hospitals have increased their income by establishing international departments.

CD 2-24

In Japan, remuneration to hospitals for treatment costs is
5 based on a point score set by the government. In the case of healthcare services provided by health insurance, the calculation base is set at 10 yen per point. This cost is covered jointly by health insurance and patients themselves. In the case of treatment not covered by
10 health insurance, there is no set figure for the cost per point. For example, some hospitals may set the per-point price at 30 yen while the actual cost is 10 yen. This enables hospitals to make a lot of money, because even if foreign patients receive the same medical care as
15 Japanese patients, it will not be covered by Japanese health insurance.

Generally, when foreign travelers receive medical care in Japan, they have to pay for it themselves. What is more, the unit price of medical treatment (10 yen per point)
20 must be increased to account for the extra care that foreign patients require. This includes the increased time that medical staff spend with the patients as well as costs such as medical interpretation. To help Japanese hospitals accept foreign patients, the Ministry of Health, Labor and
25 Welfare has prepared a manual and published it on the ministry's website.

CD 2-25

Medical care not covered by health insurance also includes treatments that make use of new technology. Unlike clinics that accept health insurance, institutions
30 that offer treatments that are not covered by insurance may charge higher fees. However, they may offer treatments that are more effective. New medical technology covered by medical care outside the insurance system includes unapproved anti-cancer drugs and cosmetic procedures.
35 While this kind of medical care can offer us better services, there are also risks involved. Treatment that is effective for people from one country is not necessarily suitable for patients from other countries. As a result, the

establish ／設立する

international department ／国際（診療）部

remuneration ／報酬

what is more ／そのうえ

interpretation ／通訳

The Ministry of Health, Labour and Welfare ／厚生労働省

anti-cancer drug ／抗がん剤

risk of unforeseen consequences cannot be ruled out.

unforeseen ／予定外の、不測の

Insurance-based treatments for Japanese and foreigners living in Japan require the patients to cover 30 percent of the total provided that they are enrolled in some form of
5 national health insurance. For example, if the total charge for the treatment is 100,000 yen, the patient needs to pay only 30,000 yen. However, there are legal limits set on the type and amount of medicines available under insurance-based care.

national health insurance ／国民健康保険

🎧 2-26

10 The 2020 Olympics were postponed due to the effects of the COVID-19 pandemic, which has been spreading around the world since the end of 2019. In early 2020, restrictions were implemented on entry to Japan from other countries. This led to the promotion of medical
15 tourism for medical treatment at patients' own expense being suspended. It remains to be seen how management of such medical care will be rebuilt in the future.

WPM 597語÷（読むのにかかった時間［秒］÷60）＝（　　　　　　　　）WPM

▰**Reading Comprehension**

下記の文章は、本文の内容をまとめたものです。（　）に適切な日本語を書き入れましょう。

（1.　　　　　　　　　　　）とは、自国で受けられない医療を受けに他国へ行くことです。その医療とは、がん治療などの（2.　　　　　　　　　）から（3.　　　　　　　　　）まで幅広いです。人口減少で先細りする国内の需要を補う新しい方法として、注目されています。

日本の病院の報酬は、すべての（4.　　　　　　　）に対して国が定めた（5.　　　　　）をもとにしています。日本人や、一定期間日本に住む外国人が対象となる保険診療は、患者が健康保険または（6.　　　　　　　　）の加入者であれば3割の自己負担となります。しかし、保険診療は、使用できる薬の種類・量などが決められており、法律によって制限されています。

（7.　　　　　　）の場合は1点当たりの金額を自由に設定できます。外国人旅行者が日本で医療を受ける場合、（8.　　　　　　　）の単価（1点10円）を多く費用請求することが求められています。これは、診療上の時間等が増加することや医療通訳などのコストなどを考慮するためです。自由診療では、最先端の医療技術を利用できる診療も含まれますが、（9.　　　　　　　）もあります。他国で治療結果が得られているとは言っても、自国の患者に合うかどうかは十分に実証されていないためです。また、自由診療は非常に高額です。

2019年末より世界中に感染が広がった新型肺炎の影響で、（10.　　　　　）上の活路として、自由診療の医療ツーリズムを推進する動きは止まってしまいました。これからどのように医療の経営を立て直していくのかが注目されます。

Practice Conversation 2-27

クリニックの電話での会話を聞いて、空欄にあてはまる語句を記入しましょう。
答えを確認した後、ペアになって会話を練習しましょう。

Agent : Good morning. I have a few questions about your clinic. **Is this a good time?**

Staff: **May I ask who's calling?**

Agent: My name is Lin. I am calling from a medical [1.   ] agency in China. We are hosting a group trip to Japan in April, and I was wondering if the clinic has ever [2.   ] travelers before.

Staff: Yes, we have. We offer services in minor [3.   ] [4.   ] for those clients. Would that be something they are interested in?

Agent: Yes, that's what they're looking for.

Staff: Great. We can send you quotes* for all the services we provide.

Agent: That would be great. By the way, how do we settle payments at your clinic in Japan? Do you take any international [5.   ]?

Staff: No, we don't. The payment will be out-of-pocket only. We take [6.   ] credit cards [7.   ] cash.

Agent: OK. Do you provide an [8.   ] service in Cantonese, by any chance?

Staff: Yes, we'll be able to arrange that.

Agent: Great. I think that's all my questions for now. Thank you so much for your time.

Staff: You're welcome. **Can I have your contact information** so I can send you the quotes?

----

*quote 見積もり

Useful Expressions 2-28

- **Is this a good time (to talk)?** (今お時間いただいてもよろしいでしょうか。)

- **May I ask who's calling?** (お名前をお伺いしてもよろしいでしょうか。[電話対応の際])

- **Can I have your contact information?**
  (ご連絡先をお伺いしてもよろしいでしょうか。)

Activities

病院を経営していくうえで、どこから収入を得るかを考えることは重要です。以下のシナリオに沿って、自分の意見を英語で述べましょう。

> **シナリオ：**あなたはある病院の経営企画部にいます。増加する訪日外国人に向けた診療を積極的に行うか、行わないかの立場を決めて、役員たちを説得しなければなりません。

State your opinion（自分が外国人患者の受け入れに賛成か反対か）

_____

_____

_____

Support your opinion （そのように考える理由を述べましょう）

- _____

- _____

- _____

Restate your opinion（外国人患者の受け入れに賛成か反対かを再度述べましょう）

_____

_____

_____

▶クラスメイトに向けて、あなたの意見をプレゼンテーションしましょう。プレゼンテーションを聞いたクラスメイトは、それに対して自分の意見を述べましょう。

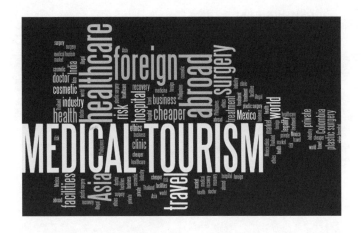

●外来受診時の診療費の領収書

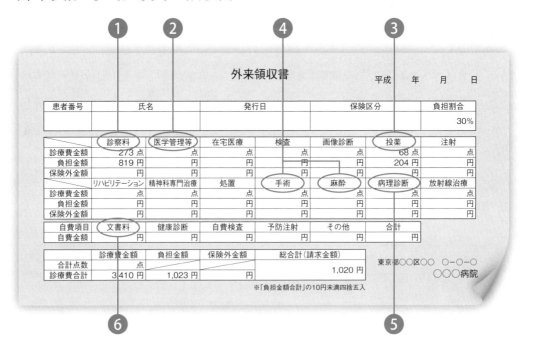

外来領収書

平成　　年　　月　　日

患者番号	氏名	発行日	保険区分	負担割合
				30%

	診察料	医学管理等	在宅医療	検査	画像診断	投薬	注射
診療費金額	273 点	点	点	点	点	68 点	点
負担金額	819 円	円	円	円	円	204 円	円
保険外金額	円	円	円	円	円	円	円
	リハビリテーション	精神科専門治療	処置	手術	麻酔	病理診断	放射線治療
診療費金額	点	点	点	点	点	点	点
負担金額	円	円	円	円	円	円	円
保険外金額	円	円	円	円	円	円	円
自費項目	文書料	健康診断	自費検査	予防注射	その他	合計	
自費金額	円	円	円	円	円	円	

	診療費金額	負担金額	保険外金額	総合計(請求金額)
合計点数	点			
診療費合計	3,410 円	1,023 円	円	1,020 円

※「負担金額合計」の10円未満四捨五入

東京都○○区○○　○−○−○
○○○病院

1	診察料	First / subsequent visit fees	診察を受けたことによる料金。初回と 2 回目以降などで変わります。検査のみのときはかかりません。
2	医学管理等	Medical supervision charges, etc.	療養上必要な管理・指導を行った際にかかります。
3	投薬	Medications	薬代・手数料のほか、処方料なども含まれます。
4	手術・麻酔	Surgery / Anesthesia	薬や医療材料以外の手術や輸血、麻酔の技術料です。
5	病理診断	Pathological diagnosis	検査、手術で採取した組織を調べる費用です。
6	文書料	Documentation fee	診断書・証明書などにかかる費用です。

●参考URL
厚生労働省：https://www.mhlw.go.jp/seisakunitsuite/bunya/kenkou_iryou/iryou/kokusai/setsumeisiryo/dl/en13.pdf
ヤマトグループ健康組合：https://www.ytckempo.or.jp/hp/shikumi/ryoushuushou.html

UNIT 12

Hopes in Regenerative Medicine

再生医療の夢

体の「若返り」や「再生」は、長い歴史上どの時代の人にとっても手の届かない憧れの対象でした。iPS 細胞の発見をはじめとする近年の科学研究と技術の成果により、自分自身の細胞をもとに必要な細胞や組織を作り、病気や老化のために失った体の機能を修復する技術が発達してきています。衰えた臓器を丸ごと交換したり、不治の病と言われていた病を治療したり、健康寿命を飛躍的に延ばしたり、という夢が叶う未来が来るのでしょうか。

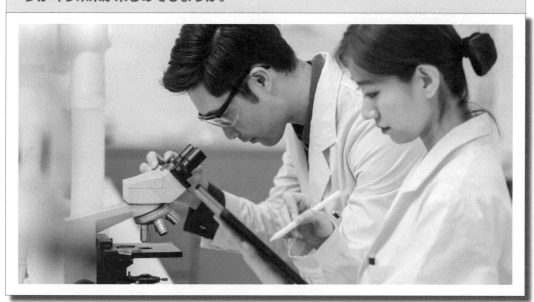

Pre-Reading Questions

ペアになり、以下について話し合いましょう。

If regenerative medicine was readily available today, what kind of treatment would you like to receive?

Vocabulary Check

次の単語とその定義を結びつけましょう。

1. generate   (a) a prolonged public disagreement
2. alleviate   (b) structural material consisting of specific cells
3. eliminate   (c) to remove something that is not needed
4. tissue   (d) to produce or create something
5. controversy   (e) to make something less severe or serious

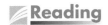
Reading

下記の英文を読みましょう。

🎧 2-29

Have you ever been amazed by the ability of a lizard to regenerate its tail after it has been lost? Have you ever thought, "It would be great if humans can do that." That may have been the thought of Aristotle, who observed
5　the phenomenon back in 330 B.C. [1] Human fascination at the idea of regeneration had been just a dream then, but it has become a reality, at least partially, in the present day, 23 centuries later.

fascination ／強い興味、魅了
regeneration ／再生

🎧 2-30

Regenerative medicine refers to a wide range of
10　technologies that involve therapies aimed at achieving the "3R's"— rejuvenation, regeneration, and replacement of damaged tissue or organ. [1][2] It includes the use of stem cells, tissue engineering, and the production of artificial organs. [1] In other words, new living cells,
15　tissues, or organs may be tailor-made in the laboratory and placed into the body to restore their lost function. Regenerative medicine has the potential to transform medical practice in a fundamental way. The focus of medical practice will shift from symptom management to curative
20　treatment. [1][2]

rejuvenation ／活性化、若返り
replacement ／交換
stem cells ／幹細胞
tissue engineering ／ヒト組織工学

symptom ／症状
curative ／治癒的な

🎧 2-31

The recent remarkable progress in regenerative medicine has been accelerated by two major factors. One is the strong demand for alleviating the high socioeconomic burden of the global aging population. [1][2][3] The world is
25　seeking more effective, economically sustainable therapies for health problems common in the elderly. They include heart disease, cancer, stroke, pulmonary disease, and diabetes [3].

sustainable ／持続可能な

pulmonary ／肺の

diabetes ／糖尿病

The other factor is the advance of new technologies including nanotechnology, bioengineering, and stem cell therapy. [1] One of the major breakthroughs was the development of induced pluripotent stem cells (iPS cells)
5 by a team led by Nobel Prize winner Professor Shinya Yamanaka. iPS cells can turn into any type of cells in the body, such as cells of the heart, nerves, and blood. In contrast to the previous method, which required taking cells from a one-week old embryo, iPS cells can be
10 generated from an adult's skin or other cells. This new method has eliminated the ethical controversy surrounding the use of human embryonic stem cells (ES cells). [4]

 2-32

Regenerative medicine may offer solutions for many conditions, whether congenital or acquired. Many clinical
15 trials are underway to find cures for various conditions that used to be thought irreversible.[1] People with diabetes may be able to have new pancreatic cells that secrete insulin properly. People with weak eyesight may be able to have new eye cells so they can see better.
20 People who had a heart attack may be able to have damaged muscles or vessels of the heart replaced with new ones.

2-33

The next step, which is a dream of many, is generating a whole organ using 3-dimensional printing technology.
25 Failure of an organ, such as the kidney or the liver, has traditionally been addressed by organ transplant therapy, in which an organ is taken from a donor.[1] If the new technology allows a patient to be his or her own donor, the issues of long waiting lists and the body's response
30 of rejecting the foreign organ may be resolved. Because organs are much larger and more complex than cells and tissues, organ production and its real-world application have a long way to go.[4] Regenerating a whole "tail" may

nanotechnology ／ナノテクノロジー

bioengineering ／生物工学

breakthrough ／突破口

iPS cells ／人工多機能性幹細胞

nerve ／神経

embryo ／ヒトの胚

ES cells ／胚性幹細胞

acquired ／後天的な

irreversible ／不可逆の、治療不能の

pancreatic ／すい臓の

3-D printing ／３次元印刷

kidney ／腎臓

liver ／肝臓

transplant ／移植

be a dream still. However, regenerative medicine surely offers new hopes for extending healthy life expectancy, which is so vital in the light of the global aging population.

life expectancy／寿命

1. Transforming Healthcare through Regenerative Medicine, BMC Medicine, 2016
2. The Regenerative Horizon: Opportunities for Nursing Research and Practice, Journal of Nursing Scholarship, 2019
3. Regenerative Medicine: Transforming the Drug Discovery and Development Paradigm, Cold Spring Harbor Perspectives in Medicine, 2014
4. What Are iPS Cells? Center for iPS Cell Research and Application, 2020

WPM 552語÷(読むのにかかった時間[秒]÷60) = (　　　　　　　　　　)WPM

◤Reading Comprehension

下記の表は、本文の内容をまとめたものです。(　)に入る適切な英単語を語群から選び記入しましょう。

What is regenerative medicine?	Technologies that involve therapies aimed at the "3R's"— (1.　　　　　　　), (2.　　　　　　　　), and (3.　　　　　　　) of damaged cells and tissues.
What is accelerating the progress in regenerative medicine?	The strong demand for alleviating the (4.　　　　　　) burden of diseases common in the (5.　　　　　　). The advance in nanotechnology, bioengineering, and (6.　　　　　　) cell therapy.
What are iPS cells?	Stem cells that can be generated from adult (7.　　　　　　) cells.
What are ES cells?	Stem cells that can be taken from an (8.　　　　　　).
What is the future goal of regenerative medicine?	Generating a whole (9.　　　　　　) using 3-dimensional printing technology.

語　　群
regeneration / controversy / recession / replacement / removal / socioeconomic / psychological / tissue / organ / skin / embryo / ethical / renovation / rejuvenation / disabled / elderly / stem / recovery

Practice Conversation 2-34

クリニックの電話での会話を聞いて、空欄にあてはまる語句を記入しましょう。
答えを確認した後、ペアになって会話を練習しましょう。

Staff: (Phone rings) ABC Clinic. **How may I help you?**

Patient: Hi, I'm traveling to Japan next month, and I have some questions about the services [1.   ] at your clinic.

Staff: Sure. We offer therapies to improve health using [2.   ] medical technologies. They are done to [3.   ] cells in the body, [4.   ] it is for disease prevention, healing, or anti-aging.

Patient: Yes, I saw that on your website. How are those therapies done?

Staff: We take cells from your fat tissue and send them to a special [5.   ]. After a few weeks, we put the newly [6.   ] cells into your body [7.   ] IV drips.

Patient: I see. So, I would be using my own cells to heal my body then.

Staff: Exactly. **Have you ever had any major illnesses before?**

Patient: Yes, I had liver cancer a few years ago. It was treated successfully. I don't have any [8.   ] right now, but I would like to try the therapy to stay well.

Staff: I see. Would you like to make an appointment with our doctor to discuss some options?

Patient: That would be great.

Useful Expressions 2-35

- **How may I help you?**（[電話を受ける際の言葉]もしもし。/ どうされましたか。）

- **Have you ever had any major illnesses before?**
  （過去に大きな病気になったことはありますか。）

Writing Tips

Persuasive Expression

説得力のある文章を書くには、説得力のある構成や言葉遣いが重要です。構成は、最初に主張を述べて理由で主張を支持します。言葉遣いは、たとえば動詞を選ぶときには、英語のPhrasal Verb（動詞＋前置詞、例えば、carry out）を使うより、ラテン語起源の動詞(例えば、implement)を用いるようにすると、知的な印象を与えることができます。堂々とした態度や目をそらさないなどの非言語的コミュニケーションも重要です。日本語にも言えることですが、直接「これがいい！」とゴリ押しのように主張するだけでは、納得してもらうのが難しいです。あくまでも客観的に、説得したいことを行う利点を3つ程度に絞って提示します。本当に大切なことは、繰り返し述べることで相手の印象に残ります。

Activities

再生医療の技術を用いた治療は、国内でもすでに行われており、日々その活躍の場が広がっていますが、まだ誰にでも手の届く治療というわけではありません。以下のシナリオに沿って、英語で意見を述べましょう。

> **シナリオ：**あなたは議員です。超高齢化を背景に、再生医療技術の需要が高まっていますが、費用が高いため、保険適用にすべきだとの国民の声が高まっています。再生医療技術を用いた治療の中で、優先的に健康保険の適用 (covered by insurance) にすべき分野について、熱い議論が交わされています。あなたは次の **Option A〜D** について、どの分野を優先すべきか、会議で意見を発表することになりました。

Option A. Cancer therapies がん免疫細胞療法など

Option B. Dental therapies：口腔内組織と骨の再生など

Option C. Skin therapies 皮膚の再生、創傷治癒など

Option D. Joint disease therapies 関節、筋肉、腱、靭帯の損傷や変性の治療など

State the problem (現在の問題を述べましょう)

_____

_____

_____

▼

State your opinion (あなたの意見を述べましょう)

_____

_____

_____

▼

Support your opinion (その意見が賢明だと思う理由を述べましょう)

● _____

● _____

● _____

▼

Restate your opinion (あなたの結論を再度述べましょう)

_____

_____

_____

▶クラスメイトを会議の参加者と想定して、あなたの意見を発表しましょう。発表を聞い
　たクラスメイトは、意見に対して一言自分の感想を英語で述べましょう。

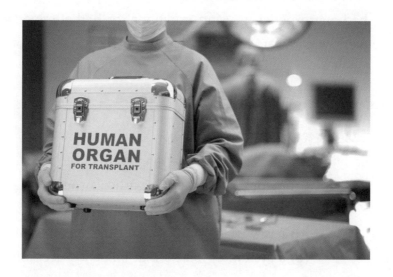

Traditional Medicine in the Modern World

現代における伝統医療

伝統医療に対してどんなイメージを持っていますか。中国医学やアーユルヴェーダ医学などを代表とする伝統医療は、それぞれの地域で長い年月をかけて培われてきました。世界中で西洋医学がスタンダードとして受け入れられ、多くの国では長らく「根拠がない」と表舞台から退いていたように思われる伝統医療ですが、近年ではその哲学が広く受け入れられ、伝統医療も含めた多種多様な選択肢を求める患者が増えています。伝統医療と従来型の医療はうまく共存できるのでしょうか。

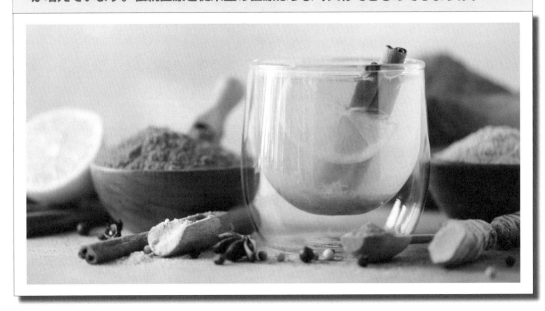

Pre-Reading Questions

ペアになり、以下について話し合いましょう。

Have you had any experience using traditional or herbal remedies at home when you were sick? What was your experience like?

Vocabulary Check

次の単語とその定義を結びつけましょう。

1. compliant   (a) certain that something is true
2. philosophy   (b) made just right for a particular need
3. expertise   (c) an opinion of an expert
4. tailored   (d) easily willing to do what other people want
5. convinced   (e) a system of beliefs that influence decisions or actions

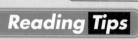

Topic Study

ある特定のテーマに関する英文を読み書きする際には、まずそのテーマの中でよく使用される単語の意味や概念、スタイルを日英両方で調べてから読み書きすると、スムーズに進みます。伝統医療や医療の歴史に関する英文を読む場合は、まずそのトピックに関してインターネットなどで調べて、関連する日本語の文章を読んでから英文を読むとわかりやすくなります。

▰Reading

下記の英文を読みましょう。

 2-36

Fernando is a young, healthy, and educated man from Sri Lanka working in Japan. One day he visited a doctor as he suddenly developed an unusually high fever, body aches, and coughing. Dr. Sato diagnosed him with
5 influenza and prescribed Fernando a course of medicine. Fernando was relieved to know that it was not something more serious and told her that he would be fine without the medicine. He also told her that he had brought a special tea from back home that he knew worked better
10 than regular medicine. Dr. Sato felt slightly offended as she thought her expertise was being ignored. She told Fernando that such tea would not work. Fernando also felt slightly offended because she seemed to disrespect a tradition so important to his native culture. Of course,
15 the doctor is more knowledgeable in the field of medicine. But is this matter as simple as Fernando being a "non-compliant" patient? The answer lies in the fact that different paradigms of medicine exist in the world.

offended ／気分を害した

paradigm ／枠組み、パラダイム

🎧 2-37

Many agree that Hippocrates (460-377 B.C.) of Greece was the "father of modern medicine." Prior to his time, illnesses were handled mainly by temple priests through spiritual practices. He believed that nature has the ability
5 to heal the human body and treated patients with herbs, proper diet, exercise, and lifestyle changes. Hippocratic medicine lasted as the main form of medicine in the western world for a remarkably long time, until the 1500s. Around that time, Paracelsus (1493-1541 A.D.) of
10 Switzerland introduced a different idea. He believed that the human body can be healed by the use of minerals, as opposed to plants in Hippocratic medicine. Inspired by alchemy and astronomy, he emphasized the importance of chemistry in medicine. It is said that
15 conventional medicine of today, which largely relies on pharmacotherapy, is the successor of Paracelsus's approach.[1]

🎧 2-38

So-called "traditional" medicine today refers to forms of medicine outside conventional medicine, which uses pharmacotherapy, surgery, and radiation as its main
20 therapies.[2] Throughout history, many cultures of the world have developed their own unique systems of maintaining health. Perhaps the most well-known examples are Traditional Chinese Medicine and Indian Ayurvedic Medicine, with thousands of years of history. [3]
25 Interestingly, those traditional medicines share a common philosophy. They focus on health rather than disease, aim to find a balance between mind, body, and environment, and use plants as remedies. [4]

🎧 2-39

Traditional forms of medicine had been generally ignored
30 in medical settings in the industrialized world, as they lacked evidence from scientific research. In recent decades, however, traditional medicine has been steadily gaining in popularity. One reason may be that it is more affordable. Another reason may be that the philosophy
35 behind it has become more popular. Increasing concerns

mineral ／鉱物

alchemy ／錬金術
astronomy ／天文学
conventional ／従来型の
pharmacotherapy ／薬物療法
successor ／継承者

Traditional Chinese Medicine ／伝統中国医学

Indian Ayurvedic Medicine ／インドのアーユルヴェーダ医学

remedy ／治療薬

steadily ／着実に

about the adverse effects of synthetic medicines may also be a contributing factor. [4] Whatever the reason, people now desire tailored care chosen from as many options as possible. Healthcare providers, on the other hand, may be more cautious as interactions with conventional therapies can be dangerous or mostly unknown.

In the example earlier, the doctor and the patient were both convinced they knew the "right thing to do." The doctor was following one paradigm of medicine. The patient, as with many people today, wanted to choose from options across different paradigms of medicine. The patient wanted the conventional diagnostic testing and the traditional herbal remedy at the same time.

🎧 2-40

To bridge the gap between the two, a new field of medicine called "integrative medicine" has emerged. Clinicians trained in integrative medicine make the best use of both worlds. They neither reject conventional medicine nor accept traditional medicine without carefully investigating evidence regarding its efficacy and safety. In integrative medicine, clinicians and patients work together as partners to facilitate the body's innate ability to heal itself. They use both conventional and non-conventional therapies to achieve better health. [5] Integrative medicine seems to be a happy marriage between evidence-based practice and long-valued tradition. Will this marriage stay strong? Will it be the next form of "conventional medicine"? You will be the one to find out.

1. Back to Eden, Jethro Kloss, 2004
2. Conventional Medicine, National Cancer Institute, 2020
3. Wellness and Prevention, Johns Hopkins Medicine, 2020
4. Herbal Medicine: Biomolecular and Clinical Aspects 2nd Edition, Benzie et al., 2011
5. The Defining Principles of Integrative Medicine, The University of Arizona, 2020

Glossary (margin notes):

- adverse effect ／副作用
- synthetic medicine ／合成薬
- interaction ／相互作用
- integrative medicine ／統合医療
- efficacy ／効果
- facilitate ／促進する
- innate ／持って生まれた

WPM 673語÷（読むのにかかった時間[秒]÷60）＝（　　　　　　）WPM

Reading Comprehension

下記の英文を読み、本文の内容に合っているものにはT、誤っているものにはFを記入しましょう。

1. Hippocrates is famous for promoting spiritual practices as mainstream medicine in the Western world for a remarkably long time. ____

2. Paracelsus believed that nature has the ability to heal the human body and treated patients with herbs, proper diet, exercise, and lifestyle changes. ____

3. Interactions between conventional medicines and traditional remedies can be dangerous or mostly unknown. ____

4. Most patients and healthcare providers desire treatment options chosen from different paradigms of medicine. ____

5. Patients who do not follow instructions based on conventional medicine should always be considered as non-compliant patients. ____

6. Medical professionals trained in integrative medicine neither reject conventional medicine nor accept traditional medicine without carefully investigating evidence. ____

Practice Conversation

🎧 2-41

薬局での会話を聞いて、空欄にあてはまる語句を記入しましょう。
答えを確認した後、ペアになって会話を練習しましょう。

Pharmacist: Here are your medications. Please take this one [1.   ] an empty stomach twice a day. Please take the other one as [2.   ] for pain.

Patient: OK, thanks.

Pharmacist: **Are you taking any medications right now?**

Patient: No, but I'm taking some herbal [3.   ] prescribed by my Chinese medical doctor. Will that be a problem?

Pharmacist: Well, it could be a concern. In most cases, [4.   ] with [5.   ] medicines are unknown. Do you have them [6.   ] you?

Patient: Yes, hold on.....Here they are.

Pharmacist: I see...

Patient: My Chinese doctor told me that they are good for my [7.   ]. If possible, I would like to keep [8.   ] them.

Pharmacist: OK. **Can you give me a few minutes?** I'll look them up and see if there is likely to be a problem.

Patient: That would be great. Thank you so much.

Useful Expressions

 2-42

- **Are you taking any medications right now?**（現在お薬は飲まれていますか。）

- **Can you give me a few minutes?**（数分お時間をいただけますか。）

Activities

伝統医療は、それぞれの地域で長い年月をかけて培われてきた大切な文化です。健康や病気に対して多種多様な考え方があることを意識することは、医療の現場において役立ちます。ペアまたはグループで、興味のある国または地域を選び、その土地に根づいている伝統医療について調べ、下の表に英語でまとめましょう。

国または地域	
伝統医療の名称	
哲学や思想	
治療の例	

表でまとめた情報をもとに、クラスで英語で発表しましょう。

In our group, we looked at a traditional form of medicine called ＿＿＿＿＿＿＿
（伝統医療の名称）in ＿＿＿＿＿＿＿＿＿＿＿＿＿（国名）.

They believe that

＿＿＿＿＿＿＿＿＿＿＿＿＿＿＿＿＿＿＿＿＿＿＿＿＿＿＿＿＿＿＿＿＿＿＿＿

＿＿＿＿＿＿＿＿＿＿＿＿＿＿＿＿＿＿＿＿＿＿＿＿＿＿＿＿＿＿＿＿＿＿＿＿

＿＿＿＿＿＿＿＿＿＿＿＿＿＿＿＿＿＿＿＿＿＿＿＿＿＿＿＿＿＿＿＿＿＿＿＿

＿＿＿＿＿＿＿＿＿＿＿＿＿＿＿＿＿＿＿＿＿＿＿＿＿＿＿＿＿＿＿＿＿＿＿＿

＿＿＿＿＿＿＿＿＿＿＿＿＿＿＿＿＿＿＿＿＿＿＿＿＿＿＿＿＿＿（哲学や思想）.

We would like to share an example of this kind of treatment.

＿＿＿＿＿＿＿＿＿＿＿＿＿＿＿＿＿＿＿＿＿＿＿＿＿＿＿＿＿＿＿＿＿＿＿＿

＿＿＿＿＿＿＿＿＿＿＿＿＿＿＿＿＿＿＿＿＿＿＿＿＿＿＿＿＿＿＿＿＿＿＿＿

＿＿＿＿＿＿＿＿＿＿＿＿＿＿＿＿＿＿＿＿＿＿＿＿＿＿＿＿＿＿＿＿＿＿＿＿

＿＿＿＿＿＿＿＿＿＿＿＿＿＿＿＿＿＿＿＿＿＿＿＿＿＿＿＿＿＿＿＿＿＿＿＿

＿＿＿＿＿＿＿＿＿＿＿＿＿＿＿＿＿＿＿＿＿＿＿＿＿＿＿＿＿＿＿＿＿＿＿＿

Thank you for listening. Do you have any questions?

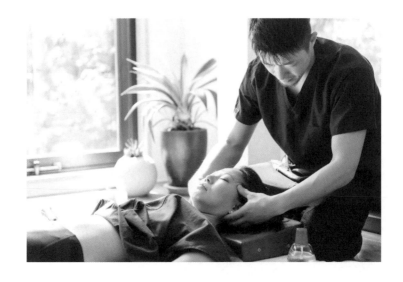

Japan's Healthcare System Is the Envy of the World

世界がうらやむ日本の医療制度

日本の国民皆保険制度は、世界でも類を見ない理想的な医療保険制度です。私たちが普段当たり前に享受している保険制度について、改めて考えてみましょう。

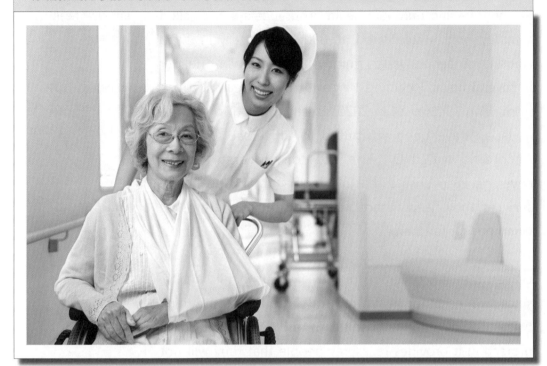

Pre-Reading Questions

ペアになり、以下について話し合いましょう。

What would you do if you were not covered by any insurance?

Vocabulary Check

次の単語とその定義を結びつけましょう。

1. attribute	**(a)**	the effect that something has on another thing
2. uninsured	**(b)**	not covered by insurance
3. impact	**(c)**	the fact of no longer developing or making progress
4. stagnation	**(d)**	without enough money to pay what you owe
5. bankrupt	**(e)**	to believe that something is the result of a particular thing

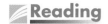
Reading

下記の英文を読みましょう。

🎧 2-43

Japanese live longer than Americans despite spending only half as much on health care. Many rely on the inexpensive and universal health insurance system, called *kaihoken*, which celebrated its 60th anniversary in 2021.

5 During this period, Japan quickly became a world leader in several fields, including longevity. Life expectancy rose from 52 in 1945 to 84 in 2020. Excellent health outcomes in Japan have been attributed to universal coverage. According to WHO, "The goal of universal health

10 coverage is to ensure that all people obtain the health services they need without suffering financial hardship when paying for them."

🎧 2-44

Universal health coverage directly impacts public health, since high costs for health care might make people think

15 twice about visiting a hospital. In addition, the financial protection it provides reassures people that they will not be impoverished or bankrupted by having to pay large health care bills out of their own pocket. Seen in this context, universal health coverage is one of the main

20 pillars of a sustainable society as well as a vital part of any effort to reduce social inequities.

🎧 2-45

Depicting the underlying reasons for Japan's success in health care works as a role model for other nations looking to achieve good outcomes at affordable cost.

25 Japan's approach to achieving universal health coverage, which rests on establishing a form of social health insurance that is both employee-based (*shakaihoken*)and community-based (*kokuminhoken*), has advantages but

universal health insurance system ／国民皆保険

longevity ／長寿
life expectancy ／寿命

suffer ／苦しむ

bankrupt ／破産する、経済的に破綻する

inequity ／不均衡、不公平

affordable ／許容できる

also drawbacks. On the plus side, as a result of the National Insurance Law being amended in 1961 to establish a universal health insurance system (*kaihoken*), almost everyone is now insured. The application of the
5 same fee schedule across these two plans and all healthcare providers has ensured equity and kept costs at a reasonable level, and the co-payment rate of 30 percent is the same for everyone apart from senior citizens and children. These equitable results have been
10 achieved thanks to state subsidies to plans that enroll people with lower incomes. On the negative side, the fragmentation of enrollment into different plans has led to some people being charged three times as much as others in the proportion of their income paid as
15 premiums, as well as the growing problem of an uninsured population. What is more, Japan's birthrate has been declining in recent years and the population is aging, leading to an increase in medical expenses. Since maintaining the system relies on public funds, this
20 increase has become a significant burden on national finances.

co-payment rate ／自己負担率

premium ／掛け金、保険料

🎧 2-46

Some problems lie ahead for Japan's *kaihoken* system. Although it needs a growing workforce to pay the bills, Japan is aging and its population is shrinking. Since
25 *kaihoken* was established in 1961, the proportion of people over 65 has quadrupled, to 28 percent of the population. By 2050 it will be two-fifths of the population. "The Japanese health system that had worked in the past has begun to fail," Kenji Shibuya, professor at University
30 of London, King's College London, and other experts write in a British medical journal, devoted to *kaihoken*. "The system's inefficiencies could be tolerated in a period of high growth, but not in today's climate of economic stagnation."

quadruple ／ 4 倍の、4者間の

Still, it is true that Japan's universal healthcare system is a target of envy from other countries. The Japanese should be justly proud of their healthcare system. People get good basic care and are never bankrupted by medical
5 bills.

WPM 563語÷(読むのにかかった時間[秒]÷60) = (　　　　　　　　　　)WPM

▨ Reading Comprehension

下記の文章は、本文の内容をまとめたものです。(　)に適切な日本語を書き入れましょう。

日本人が良好な健康状態で生活できるのは、(1.　　　　　　　　　) のおかげです。それは人々の健康に直接的な影響を与えてきました。もしも (2.　　　　　　) が高すぎれば、人々は病院に行こうとは思わないかもしれません。また、経済的負担から人々を守ることにより、人々が自費で医療費を払うことで (3.　　　　　) 化するのを防ぐことができます。国民皆保険はこのように (4.　　　　　　) な社会の発展に不可欠な要素であり、(5.　　　　　　) を減らすための重要な要素なのです。日本の皆保険制度には問題もあります。医療費を払う労働人口を増やす必要があるのにもかかわらず、日本は (6.　　　　　) 化しておりその (7.　　　　) は減少しています。それでもなお、日本の皆保険制度は他国からみて羨望の的であることは事実です。日本はこの医療制度を誇りに思うべきです。人々は良い基本的なケアを受けることができて、医療費により (8.　　　　　　　　　　　) ことがないのですから。

▨ Practice Conversation

内科の受付での会話を聞いて、空欄にあてはまる語句を記入しましょう。
答えを確認した後、ペアになって会話を練習しましょう。

Patient: Excuse me. Is this the reception for Internal Medicine?

Staff: Yes, it is. May I help you?

Patient: Yes. I've [1.　　　] this cold for two weeks, and I just need to have something [2.　　　　　] by a doctor.

Staff: I see. Do you have your insurance card?

Patient: Here it is. Does this insurance [3.　　　　] my visit today? I just moved to Japan last month, and I don't really know how it works.

Staff: It does, but you will have to pay a [4.　　　　　　　].

Patient: Oh, I didn't know that. Can you give me an idea of how much?

Staff: It'll be about 30 percent of the total cost. A few thousand yen [5.   ] be enough for a visit and medication in the case of a cold, for example.

Patient: That sounds pretty [6.   ]. I'm glad I'm [7.   ].

Staff: Since this is your first visit, **can you please fill out this form?**

Patient: Sure.

Staff: **Please have a seat**. We'll call your name [8.   ]. **Please let me know if you have any questions**.

Patient: OK. Thank you for your help.

Useful Expressions

 2-49

- **Can you please fill out this form?**（この用紙に記入していただけますか。）

- **Please have a seat.**（どうぞおかけください。）

- **Please let me know if you have any questions.**
（何かわからないことがあれば声をかけてください。）

Writing Tips

Logical Expansion

日本語で説明や報告をするとき、細かい状況を説明し、背景を十分に話した後に結論を書くと理解してもらえると思います。それは日本語の論理展開です。日本語には日本語の、英語には英語の論理展開があり、意見を述べたり書いたりするときには、その言語の論理展開に従わないと理解してもらえないことがあります。英語では先に「結論」を述べ、その結論を支持する理由を列挙するのが一般的な論理の展開方法です。日本語のように起承転結で述べて結論を最後まで書かないということがないようにしましょう。

Activities

世界でも珍しい日本の国民皆保険ですが、それを実施する際の、メリット・デメリットはどのようなものでしょうか。個人で保険に入る場合と比較して、それぞれのメリット・デメリットを下の表に英語で記入しましょう。

	Advantage	Disadvantage
Take out private insurance		
Universal coverage		

▶作文したことを、グループで発表しましょう。クラスメイトが発表したら、それに対して英語で一言意見を言いましょう。

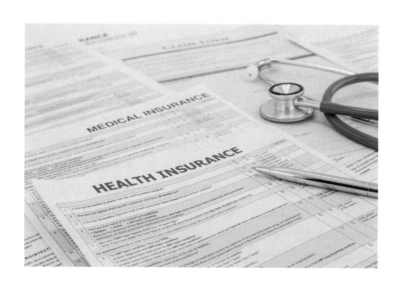

国民皆保険制度の意義

● 我が国は、国民皆保険制度を通じて世界最高レベルの平均寿命と保健医療水準を実現。
● 今後とも現行の社会保険方式による国民皆保険を堅持し、国民の安全・安心な暮らしを保証していくことが必要。

日本の国民皆保険制度の特徴

❶ 国民全員を公的医療保険で保障。

❷ 医療機関を自由に選べる。（フリーアクセス）

❸ 安い医療費で高度な医療。

❹ 社会保険方式を基本としつつ、皆保険を維持するため、公費を投入。

日本の国民医療費の負担構造（財源別）

※平成29年度

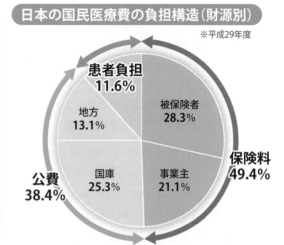

患者負担 11.6%
地方 13.1%
被保険者 28.3%
公費 38.4%
国庫 25.3%
事業主 21.1%
保険料 49.4%

我が国の医療提供体制の概略

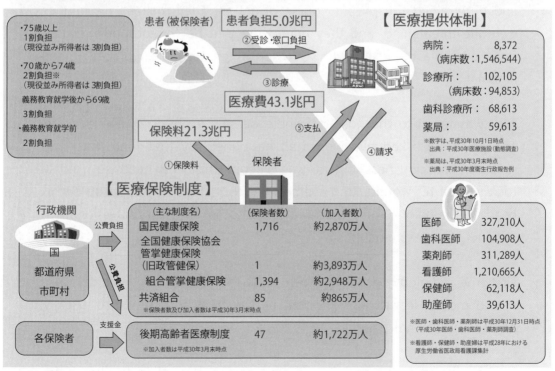

・75歳以上
1割負担
（現役並み所得者は3割負担）

・70歳から74歳
2割負担※
（現役並み所得者は3割負担）
義務教育就学後から69歳
3割負担

・義務教育就学前
2割負担

患者（被保険者）　患者負担5.0兆円
②受診・窓口負担
③診療
医療費43.1兆円
⑤支払
④請求

保険料21.3兆円
①保険料　保険者

【医療提供体制】

病院：　　　　　8,372
（病床数：1,546,544）
診療所：　　　102,105
（病床数：94,853）
歯科診療所：　68,613
薬局：　　　　59,613
※数字は、平成30年10月1日時点
出典：平成30年医療施設（動態調査）
※薬局は、平成30年3月末時点
出典：平成30年度衛生行政報告例

【医療保険制度】

行政機関
国
都道府県
市町村

各保険者

公費負担
公費負担
支援金

（主な制度名）	（保険者数）	（加入者数）
国民健康保険	1,716	約2,870万人
全国健康保険協会管掌健康保険（旧政管健保）	1	約3,893万人
組合管掌健康保険	1,394	約2,948万人
共済組合	85	約865万人

※保険者数及び加入者数は平成30年3月末時点

後期高齢者医療制度	47	約1,722万人

※加入者数は平成30年3月末時点

医師　　　　327,210人
歯科医師　　104,908人
薬剤師　　　311,289人
看護師　　1,210,665人
保健師　　　62,118人
助産師　　　39,613人

※医師・歯科医師・薬剤師は平成30年12月31日時点
（平成30年医師・歯科医師・薬剤師調査）
※看護師・保健師・助産婦は平成28年における
厚生労働省医政局看護課集計

厚生労働省「我が国の医療保険について」より引用
http://www.mhlw.go.jp/stf/seisakunitsuite/bunya/kenkou_iryou/iryouhoken/iryouhoken01/index.html

Test Your Reading Skill : Team Medicine

チーム医療

これまで、多くの英文を読んできました。最後にあなたの今の単語力と、英文をどれだけ速く正確に読む力があるかをもう一度測定しましょう。勉強を始める前と比べて、上達しているでしょうか。確かめてみましょう。

方法

1. 携帯電話や時計のストップウォッチ機能を起動します。
2. 先生の、「始め」という合図とともに読み始めましょう。
3. 読み終えたら、読むのにかかった時間を記録しましょう。
4. 本文の後の問題に答えましょう。
5. 最後に、もう一度最初から読んで、本文中のわからない単語に○を付けてください。

 2-50

Toru was a naughty 10-year-old boy. One day, when he was climbing a tree with his friends, he saw a big insect crawling on it. He yelled and he fell down from the tree. His friends laughed at him, but gradually they became anxious because he did not open his eyes or even move. They called an ambulance, and paramedics rushed to the scene and took Toru to a nearby hospital. The paramedics quickly assessed the situation and determined the proper course of action. They realized his injuries were life-threatening, and they made sure that he was properly secured on a portable medical table stretcher which they then placed in the ambulance.

 2-51

Toru was taken to the hospital, where he saw a physician and a nurse. The physician asked him what had happened. By that time, Toru had regained consciousness, but he was bleeding from his head, so a nurse took care of his wound. Toru seemed fine, but since he had fallen on his head from a height, the physician directed other medical professionals to conduct some examinations.

First, the radiology technician took an X-ray. It was very hard for Toru not to move. He was also shocked by the flash and the noise. Luckily, however, it was not painful.

He had blood taken and it was sent to the clinical technologist for analysis. The clinical technologist plays a crucial role in the process of detecting, identifying, and diagnosing illnesses and diseases. As a result of the X-ray and the blood test, no abnormality was found. To make sure, Toru was sent to an orthoptist for an eye test. Orthoptists help physicians to diagnose and treat a range of eye conditions. They carry out tests to help physicians to diagnose problems and determine appropriate treatment.

The results of the eye test were normal. Toru was discharged from the hospital but was told to visit periodically for physiotherapy. With the help of a physiotherapist, Toru will undergo some programs including working and moving his neck. A pharmacist will make sure if Toru understands the medications he takes.

CD 2-52

Can you count how many kinds of medical professionals helped Toru? In this passage, there were eight, but, many other care providers play a role in a patient's health.

Every day, these medical professionals work together and discuss each patient's progress. In this way, everyone on the care team can update the care plan along with the patient.

CD 2-53

Working as part of a team can come as something of a shock to experienced medical professionals. In their normal practice, they are accustomed to a strictly top-down approach, with the doctor making the decision and instructing a team of professionals to carry it out. It is only natural for experienced physicians to take a sense of pride in their knowledge, skills, and ability to set goals in patient care. But when working as part of a team, they must be prepared to set these factors aside and accept that the final decisions will be taken not individually but through consensus, the will of the majority, and deferring to those with greater expertise. But using multiple eyes can reveal many problems that could not be uncovered by a single eye. Everyone is a valuable member of the patient's care team. Respecting each other's opinions may be complex, but ultimately it is the most effective way to find the best care for the patient.

1 下記の表は、本文に出てきた職種をまとめたものです。空欄に適切な日本語を入れましょう。

職　種	仕　事　内　容
1.	
2.	
3.	
4.	
5.	
6.	
7.	
8.	

2 あなたが現在、1分間に読める文字数（WPM：words per minute）を求めましょう。
568語÷（読むのにかかった時間[秒]÷60）=（　　　　　　　　）WPM

3 ○を付けた未知の単語を見てみましょう。1行に何個ありましたか。

4 読み方を自己評価しましょう。英文を読むときに、下記のことを頭に置いて読んでいましたか。
当てはまる場合には○を、当てはまらない場合には×を（　　　）に記入しましょう。
① 主語と述語を意識していた。　　　　　　　　　　　　　（　　　）
② 最も重要な情報が何かを理解できた。　　　　　　　　　（　　　）
③ 接続詞など、意味を左右する言葉に気を付けて読めた。　（　　　）

5 Pre-test の目標の達成度と、このテキストを学習し始めてから上達したことを、英語で書きましょう

6 友人と見せ合い、発表し合いましょう。

接頭辞・接尾辞

医学用語は、意味の核となる語根に、前につく接頭辞や後ろにつく接尾辞を組み合わせたものが多いです。この構造を知っておくと、知らない単語に出会ったときに、おおよその意味を予測できます。例えば、Hepatoma という単語は、Hepat（肝臓：接頭辞）と Oma（がん：接尾辞）の組み合わせです。

医学英語の基本構造は、接頭辞 ＋ 語根（＋連結母音 O）＋接尾辞です。
（例）Gastroenterology = Gastr（接頭辞で胃の意味）＋連結母音 O+enter（語根で入るの意味）＋連結母音 O+logy（接尾辞で〜学の意味）

接頭辞 ＋ 語根のみ、語根 ＋ 接尾辞のみのこともあります。
（例）Hepatoma = Hepat+ 接尾辞 oma
（例）Hypertension =接頭辞 Hyper+tension
接頭辞が後ろに来ることはなく、接尾辞が前にくることもありません。
連結母音 O は、Hepatoma の oma のように、接尾辞が母音で始まるときには省略します。
また、Hypertension のように接頭辞を語根につなぐときにも、連結母音 O は省略します。
次の表は、医学英語を学ぶときに、まず覚えておきたい語根、接頭辞、接尾辞 100 個です。
覚えると語彙が大きく広がり、初めて見た単語でも、意味を予想することが出来ます。

頻出接頭辞、接尾辞

接 頭 辞			
1	a	否定	anemia：貧血
2	acro	先端、末端	acrosclerosis：先端硬化症
3	adeno	腺	adenocarcinoma：腺癌
4	adreno	副腎	adrenocorticotropic：副腎皮質刺激性の
5	angio	血管	angiography：血管造影
6	arthro	関節	arthrosis：関節症
7	auto-	自己	autoimmune：自己免疫
8	bi	二、両	bilateral：両側性
9	blepharo	眼瞼	blepharoptosis：眼瞼下垂
10	brady	緩徐、遅い	bradycardia：徐脈
11	bronchi,broncho	気管	bronchitis：気管支炎
12	carcino	癌	carcinomatosis：癌腫症
13	cardio	心臓	cardiomegaly：心肥大
14	cent	100	century：世紀
15	cephal(o)	頭、頭部	cephalalgia：頭痛
16	chondr(o)	軟骨	chondrosis：軟骨症
17	chromato, chromo	色、色素	chromatosome：染色体
18	contra	反対、逆	contralateral：反対側性の

19	cranio	頭蓋	craniocele：頭蓋瘤
20	cut(i)	皮膚	cutaneous：皮膚の
21	cysto	嚢、膀胱	cystoma：嚢腫
22	cyto	細胞	cytodiagnosis：細胞診
23	derma,dermo	皮膚	dermatitis：皮膚炎
24	dis	否定	disappear：消える
25	dys	困難、不全、不良	dysfunction：機能異常
26	encephalo	脳	encephalopathy：脳症、脳障害
27	endo	内部、内	endoscope：内視鏡
28	entero	腸	enterogastritis：胃腸炎
29	epi	上、上方	epiderm：表皮
30	erythro	赤	erythrocyte：赤血球
31	esophago	食道	esophagoscopy：食道鏡検査
32	fibro	線維	fibrosis：線維症
33	gastro	胃	gastroptosis：胃下垂
34	gingiv(o)	歯肉	gingivalgia：歯肉痛
35	hemato, hemo	血液	hematology：血液学
36	hemi	半分	hemisphere：半球
37	hepato	肝	hepatology：肝臓学
38	homo	同	homogeneity：均質性
39	hyper	高い、過度	hypertension：高血圧
40	hypo	低い、低下	hypotension：低血圧
41	lacti, lacto	乳	lactose：乳糖
42	mal	不良	malignant：悪性の
43	pan	全般	pandemic：流行
44	para	傍、対、副、疑似	parathyroid：副甲状腺
45	per	通して	percutaneous：経皮
46	peri	周囲、周辺	peripheral：周りの、末梢の
47	poly	多数	polyuria：多尿症
48	post	後	postpartum：分娩後の
49	pre	前	prenatal：出生前の
50	pseudo	偽	pseudojaundice：偽性黄疸
51	retro	後方	retrocardiac：心臓後方の
52	supra	上方	suprascapular：肩甲上の
53	tachy	急、速い	tachycardia：頻脈
54	tri	3	triceps：上腕三頭筋

接尾辞

55	-aemia, -haemia	血液（の状態）	anaemia: 貧血
56	-algia	痛み	myalgia: 筋肉痛
57	-centesis	穿刺	amniocentesis: 羊水穿刺
58	-cide	殺す	bactericide: 殺菌薬
59	-cis	切除	incision: 切開
60	-clast	破壊	osteoclast: 破骨細胞
61	-clysis	洗浄	rectoclysis: 点滴浣腸
62	-crine	分泌する	endocrine: 内分泌
63	-cyte	細胞	leukocyte: 白血球
64	-ectomy	切除	mastectomy: 乳房切除術
65	-emia	血液の状態	leucaemia: 白血病
66	-esis	の症状	agenesis: 非形成、不妊
67	-gen(e)	生じるもの	pathogen: 病原体
68	-gnosis	認識	prognosis: 予後
69	-graph	記録された絵・図	cardiograph: 心電計
70	-graphy	記録法	angiography: 血管造影法
71	-ia	(病的)状態	abasia: 歩行不能
72	-iatry	治療	psychiatry: 精神医学
73	-ism	病的状態	dwarfism: 小人症
74	-ist	〜研究者、医	pathologist: 病理医
75	-itis	炎症	arthritis: 関節炎
76	-ium	組織	pericardium: 心膜
77	-lepsy	発作	epilepsy: てんかん
78	-logist	〜研究者、医	urologist: 泌尿器科医
79	-logy	学問	biology: 生物学
80	-metry	測定法	optometry: 視力測定法, 検眼
81	-oid	〜状の	sarcoidosis: サルコイドーシス
82	-oma	腫瘍、瘤	hematoma: 血腫
83	-opsy	検査	biopsy: 生検
84	-osis	病的状態	osteoporosis: 骨粗しょう症
85	-pathy	病気	neuropathy: 神経障害
86	-penia	不足	osteopenia: 骨減少
87	-phagia,phagy	食欲	autophagy: 自食
88	-philia	傾向、病的愛好	hemophilia: 血友病
89	-phobia	恐怖	claustrophobia: 閉所恐怖症

90	-plasia	形成、発達	achondroplasia: 軟骨形成不全
91	-plasty	形成（術）	hip arthroplasty: 股関節置換（形成)術
92	-pnea	呼吸	apnea: 無呼吸
93	-sclerosis	硬化症	arteriosclerosis: 動脈硬化
94	-scope	検器	stethoscope: 聴診器
95	-scopy	検査	endoscopy: 内視鏡検査
96	-stenosis	狭窄（症）	restenosis: 再狭窄
97	-stomy	開口術	colostomy: 人工肛門形成(術)
98	-tome	切断器具	osteotome: 骨のみ
99	-tomy	切開、切除（術）	appendectomy:虫垂切除術
100	-trophy	栄養	muscular dystrophy:筋ジストロフィー

GLOSSARY

Pre / Post-test 2-54

Team Medicine

accustom／慣れる

clinical technologist／臨床検査技師

consciousness／意識

consensus／意見の一致

crawl／はう

life-threatening／命を脅かすような

naughty／悪い

orthoptist／視能訓練士

periodically／定期的に

physician／医師

physiotherapy／理学療法

Unit 1 2-55

How Food Passes Through Our Body

bile／胆汁

carbohydrate／炭水化物

churn／かき回す

crypt／地下室

enzyme／酵素

esophagus／食道

frond-like／葉っぱのような

gastric acid／胃液

gut／消化管、腸

industrial refinery／産業用製油所

lining／（胃の）内側

mucus／粘液

peristalsis／蠕動（ぜんどう）運動

saliva／唾液

stool／便

unappetizing／おいしくない

villi／絨毛（じゅうもう）

Unit 2 2-56

Coping with Cancer: Five Stages of Grief

anger／怒り

anti-cancer drug／抗がん剤

appreciate／享受する

back and forth／前後する

breast cancer／乳がん

brown rice／玄米

calm down／落ち着く

chemotherapy／化学療法

company employee／会社員

co-worker／同僚

desperate／絶望的

early-stage／早期の

eliminate／除去する

excessive／過度の

fertility／妊孕性（にんようせい：妊娠できること）

gynecologist／婦人科医

sensation like a stone rolling／ごろごろする
　　ような感触

obstetrician／産科医

oncologist／腫瘍内科医

persuade／説得する

physician／医師

reconstruction／再建

relapse／再発する

side effect／副作用

suppress／抑え込む

Unit 3 2-57

Where Medicine Meets Religion

antibiotic／抗生物質の

approve／承認する

blood transfusion／輸血

circumspect／慎重な

derive／～から由来する

fatal／致命的な

immunity／免疫

injection／注射

intricate／複雑な

intriguing／興味をそそる

invasive／侵襲的な

IV drips／静脈点滴

meningitis／髄膜炎

microorganism／微生物

pilgrimage／巡礼

preservative／保存料

respiratory／呼吸器の

secretion／分泌物

sub-Saharan／サハラ以南の

vaccination／予防接種

weakened／弱毒化した

Unit 4 2-58

Before Calling It Malpractice

adverse event／有害事象

blame game／非難合戦

by-product／副産物

crucial／極めて重要な

frontline／前線

infection／感染症

intervention／介入

lawsuit／訴訟

malpractice／医療過誤、医療ミス

negligence／義務を怠ること、過失

rash／発疹

safeguard／～を防ぐ

slip／誤り、ミス

startling／衝撃的な

statistics／統計

unintentional／故意ではない

Unit 5 2-59

How Are Drugs Developed?

absorb／吸収する

authority／当局

billion／10 億

compound／成分

cure／治す

distribute／分布する

dose／投与量

excrete／排泄する

explore／見る、調べる

in detail／詳細に

informed consent／説明と同意、同意説明文書

lucrative／もうかる

metabolize／代謝する

one by one／1 つずつ

participant／参加者

PMDA／医薬品医療機器総合機構

proceed to／～に進む

process／過程

reject／拒否する

require／必要とする

stage／段階

submit／提出する

substance／物質

susceptible／影響を受けやすい

toxic／毒の

unexpected／予期しない

volunteer／志願者

Unit 6 2-60

What Comes First when Helping Others

decompression／減圧

ergonomic／人間工学の

hazard／危険、危害

hepatitis／肝炎

hygiene／衛生

intervention／介入

laboratory technician／検査技師

needle stick injury／針刺し損傷

occupational health／労働衛生

overlook／見落とす、目をつぶる

paramedic／救急救命士

physiotherapist／理学療法士

psychiatric／精神の

psychosocial／心理社会的な

qualified／資格を満たした

shed light on／浮き彫りにする

shortage／不足

tuberculosis／結核

workforce／労働人口

Unit 7 2-61

How to Identify Reliable Health Information

allocation／割り当て

back up／支持する

benefit／利益を得る

bias／バイアス、偏り

claim／主張

distortion／歪曲

gold standard／金科玉条

health professional／医療従事者

identify／見分ける

narrative／語り

objective／客観的な

perspective／見地

qualitative study／質的研究

RCT／ランダム化比較試験

reliable／信頼できる

room／余地

source／（情報）源

take for granted／当然と思う

tempting／誘惑するような

Unit 8 2-62

What Is "Upstream" Thinking?

AED／自動体外式除細動器

cause and effect／因果、原因と結果

chronic／慢性の

context／背景

CPR／心肺機能蘇生

discipline／分野、学科、領域

effort／努力、取り組み

epidemiology／疫学

heart attack／心臓発作

investigate／調査する

ischemic heart disease／虚血性心疾患

pandemic／世界に流行している

parable／例え話

phenomenon／現象

plaque／プラーク

public health／公衆衛生学

socioeconomic／社会経済的な

stroke／脳卒中

upstream／上流

victim／犠牲者

well-being／健康で安心なこと、福利、幸福

Unit 9 2-63

Actions Speak Louder than Words

appreciate／よく理解する、感謝する

aspect／側面

attribute／特質、特性

commonality／（性質などを）共有していること

constraint／制約

counter-intuitive／直感に反した

discomfort／不快感、不快症状

encounter／出会い、接触

genuine／心からの

inappropriate／不適切な

ingenuine／不誠実な

intimidating／怯えさせるような

itinerary／旅程

mutual／相互の、共通の

rapport／ラポール、感情的な親密さ

reassurance／安心感

supposedly／建前では、恐らくは

synchronization／同期すること

walk-in／予約なしの、飛び込みの

Unit 10 2-64

Genetic Counseling as an Emerging Field

abnormality／異常

accredited／認定された

certified／認定を受けた

congenital disability／先天性障害

ethical／倫理的な

first and foremost／何よりもまず

milestone／（歴史などにおける）画期的な出来事

motive／動機

opt to／～することを選ぶ

prenatal diagnosis／出生前診断

psychological／心理的な

scientific evidence／科学的根拠

selective abortion／選択的流産

series of medical practices／一連の医療行為

violate／違反する

well-versed／精通して

Unit 11 2-65

Can Medical Tourism Be a White Knight?

anti-cancer drug／抗がん剤

as of／～の時点で

cosmetic surgery／美容整形手術

establish／設立する

growth strategy／成長戦略

International Department／国際（診療）部

interpretation／通訳

medical tourism／医療ツーリズム

national health insurance／国民健康保険

remuneration／報酬

The Ministry of Health, Labour and Welfare／厚生労働省

unforeseen／予定外の、不測の

what is more／そのうえ

Unit 12 2-66

Hopes in Regenerative Medicine

acquired／後天的な

bioengineering／生物工学

breakthrough／突破口

curative／治癒的な

diabetes／糖尿病

embryo／ヒトの胚

ES cells／胚性幹細胞

fascination／強い興味、魅了

iPS cells／人工多機能性幹細胞

irreversible／不可逆の、治療不能の

kidney／腎臓

life expectancy／寿命

liver／肝臓

nanotechnology／ナノテクノロジー

nerve／神経

pancreatic／すい臓の

pulmonary／肺の

regeneration／再生

rejuvenation／活性化、若返り

replacement／交換

stem cells／幹細胞

sustainable／持続可能な

symptom／症状

tissue engineering／ヒト組織工学

transplant／移植

3-D printing／3次元印刷

Unit 13 2-67

Traditional Medicine in the Modern World

adverse effect／副作用

alchemy／錬金術

astronomy／天文学

conventional／従来型の

efficacy／効果

facilitate／促進する

Indian Ayurvedic Medicine／インドのアーユ
　ルヴェーダ医学

innate／持って生まれた

integrative medicine／統合医療

interaction／相互作用

mineral／鉱物

offended／気分を害した

paradigm／枠組み、パラダイム

pharmacotherapy／薬物療法

remedy／治療薬

steadily／着実に

successor／継承者

synthetic medicine／合成薬

Traditional Chinese Medicine／伝統中国医学

Unit 14 2-68

*Japan's Healthcare System Is the Envy of
the World*

affordable／許容できる

bankrupt／破産する、経済的に破綻する

co-payment rate／自己負担率

inequity／不均衡、不公平

life expectancy／寿命

longevity／長寿

premium／掛け金、保険料

quadruple／4倍の、4者間の

suffer／苦しむ

universal health insurance system／国民皆
　保険

著者紹介

大野 直子（Naoko Ono）
東京都出身。The University of Bath 修士課程（通訳翻訳学修士）、東京大学医学系研究科社会医学専攻博士後期課程（医学博士）修了。通訳案内士（英語）。国内外の医療機器メーカーにて薬事申請スペシャリスト、外資系医療機器認証機関等にて通訳者・翻訳者としての経験も持つ。帝京大学医療共通教育研究センター講師（担当科目：医療英語）を経て、現在順天堂大学国際教養学部・大学院医学研究科准教授として勤務。研究分野は医療コミュニケーション、医療通訳。

ダシルヴァ石田 牧子（Makiko Ishida DaSilva）
東京都出身。Maryville College 学士課程（生物学）、Boston College Graduate School of Nursing 修士課程（看護学）修了。米国マサチューセッツ州看護師、正看護師。国内外の医療施設において看護師として外国人診療に携わり、医療通訳・翻訳、医療留学コーディネーターとしての経験も持つ。帝京大学医療共通教育研究センター助教（担当科目：医療英語）を経て、現在は国立精神・神経医療研究センター行動医学研究部研究員およびインターナショナルスクールにて小児看護に携わる。

TEXT PRODUCTION STAFF

edited by	編集
Masato Kogame	小亀 正人

English-language editing by	英文校閲
Bill Benfield	ビル・ベンフィールド

cover design by	表紙デザイン
Nobuyoshi Fujino	藤野 伸芳

text design by	本文デザイン
Nobuyoshi Fujino	藤野 伸芳

DTP by	DTP
ALIUS(Hiroyuki Kinouchi)	アリウス（木野内 宏行）

CD PRODUCTION STAFF

narrated by	吹き込み者
Howard Colefield (AmE)	ハワード・コルフィールド（アメリカ英語）
Jennifer Okano (AmE)	ジェニファー・オカノ（アメリカ英語）

Medical World Walkabout
医療の世界を見渡そう

2021年1月20日　初版発行
2024年4月5日　第4刷発行

著　者　大野 直子
　　　　ダシルヴァ石田 牧子

発 行 者　佐野 英一郎

発 行 所　株式会社 成美堂
　　　　〒101-0052　東京都千代田区神田小川町3-22
　　　　TEL 03-3291-2261　FAX 03-3293-5490
　　　　https://www.seibido.co.jp

印 刷・製 本　三美印刷株式会社

ISBN 978-4-7919-7236-4　　　　　　　Printed in Japan